THEORY
PRACTICE OF
PSYCHIATRIC CARE

P. T. DARCY
R.M.N., S.R.N., R.C.T., R.N.T., Dip.N., Cert.Ed.

Director, College of Mental Health Nursing, Belfast,
Northern Ireland
Member of, and Examiner for the Northern Ireland National Board
for Nursing, Midwifery and Health Visiting
Member of the United Kingdom Central Council for Nursing,
Midwifery and Health Visiting

Foreword by

J. J. GORMLEY
R.M.N., S.R.N., N. Admin. Cert.

Chairman of the Training Committee for the Western Area College
of Nursing, Londonderry, Northern Ireland
Director of Nursing Services, Omagh District Health and
Social Services, Northern Ireland

HODDER AND STOUGHTON
LONDON SYDNEY AUCKLAND TORONTO

MODERN NURSING SERIES

Dedication

To the patients and staff at West Cheshire Psychiatric Hospital, Chester . . . from whom I learnt so much.

To the student nurses at West Cheshire Hospital, Chester, and Tyrone and Fermanagh Hospital, Omagh, whose interest in psychiatric nursing encouraged me to write this book.

To the Reader

Since the availability of the different drugs and instructions for their prescription change frequently, readers are advised to check with an authoritative source before administering any medication.

British Library Cataloguing in Publication Data

Darcy, P. T.
   Theory and practice of psychiatric care.
   1. Psychiatric nursing
· I. Title
   610. 73'68   RC440

ISBN 0 340 26564 7

First published 1984
Second impression 1986
Copyright © 1984 P. T. Darcy

Phototypeset by Macmillan India Ltd, Bangalore

Printed and bound in Great Britain
for Hodder and Stoughton Educational,
a division of Hodder and Stoughton Ltd,
Mill Road, Dunton Green, Sevenoaks, Kent
by Biddles Ltd, Guildford and King's Lynn

Foreword

In no field of nursing are the limits of what is regarded as a basic curriculum less easily defined than in psychiatry. The student in psychiatric nursing can usefully study such diverse subjects as senility and schizophrenia, depression and drug addiction. Each condition studied can generally be complicated by any number of psycho-social factors each in turn demanding at least a basic knowledge of that factor by the nurse.

The last decade has seen a profusion of psychiatric texts emerge, many prompted by the new developments in the field of psychiatric care over the last twenty years. This momentum of change is now becoming stabilised and the new challenges they offered for patient management are being re-examined and refined. It is a time of sober evaluation and consolidation of all that has been learned during recent growth.

It is particularly timely, therefore, for this book to appear as it provides a reliable and complete guide for the student, from the early developments right through to modern concepts and legislation. Specific illnesses are clearly explained and nursing skills are described and discussed in detail, as are the more recent developments and extensions of the nursing role. Jargon is meticulously avoided and no technique left unexplained.

The book will be welcomed by students in psychiatry and other nurses will find it a useful and comprehensive reference. Those returning to nursing after an absence will find it an easy, readable guide to enable them to relate to psychiatric nursing as it is today.

J. J. Gormley

Preface

The content and layout of this book reflect the views of 206 psychiatric student nurses. The needs they expressed arose from the practical problems encountered when caring for patients on the ward, as well as from the demands of statutory syllabuses, examinations and assessments.

The students whose challenge spurred me to write *Theory and Practice of Psychiatric Care* accepted my view that any activity undertaken which involves the nurse with the mentally ill (and in certain cases the physically ill) patient, must be regarded as part of their psychiatric nursing skills. The skill of psychiatric nursing is many faceted, but none of its aspects is exclusive. While the nurse is attending to a patient's problems or administering treatment, she may also be involved in forming a relationship with him: listening, reassuring, gaining his co-operation and encouraging him to help himself. This aspect of nursing re-enforces treatment and relates to the wider context of care objectives and the patient's individual physical, social and psychological needs.

To become proficient in the practice of psychiatric nursing, the nurse must learn to prevent her involvement in one activity from establishing something which may be detrimental to the success of another and hence will delay the patient's recovery. Ward and community experience will reduce the risk and it is less likely to happen if the nurse recognises her role in the caring team and relates each aspect to the treatment and nursing programme. To facilitate the nurse learner's role, it is necessary to maintain discussion and communication through ward meetings, so that the learner is aware of the overall care and treatment objectives.

Though this text is specifically written for nurses training for the mental part of the register, some of the basic skills discussed are also included in the syllabus for general nurse training. With the increase in secondment to psychiatric experience and the suggested psychiatry modules in the Briggs and EEC proposals, more emphasis is being placed on psychiatry and psychiatric nursing practice in training curricula and examinations. Nurses training for the general part of the register will find aspects of the following chapters particularly helpful: 2–6, 9–11, 17–19, 22–5, 27–8, 30, 37. It is hoped that this book will also be helpful to diploma in nursing students, nursing degree students, occupational therapists, social workers and registered nurses involved in ward teaching and assessments.

Contents

NOTE: Throughout this book the nurse is described as 'she' and the patient as 'he'. This is for clarity of style only. The author is a nurse himself and intends no slight to male members of the profession.

I

The Development of
Modern Psychiatry

Throughout history there has been a close association between growth in population and the growth of mental institutions. In London, the most densely populated area of medieval Britain, it

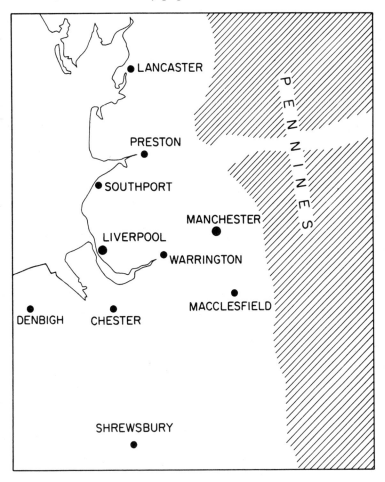

Fig. 1.1 Map to show the rapid growth of mental hospitals in populated areas within a 40 mile radius of Manchester, 1800–1850

was found necessary to open the institution later known as *Bedlam*. Originally an infirmary, it began to be used as an asylum in about 1377, its purpose being to reduce the social problem of the mentally ill, highlighted so sharply in an urban setting. There is little evidence however of other such institutions developing outside London, because of the influence of the 'manorial system' or economic unit of rural medieval Britain, and the sparsity of population. Over the following centuries the emphasis remained on community involvement through the 'parish system' or poor relief, whereby each parish helped its dependents through community effort.

Industrial approach

As the population of England continued to grow throughout the seventeenth and eighteenth centuries, the way of life was changed by the Industrial Revolution and urbanisation. This was most evident in the northern cities such as Manchester, where, in the thirty years from 1801 to 1831, the population almost trebled from 95 000 to 238 000.

Ironically, under the stress of these changes, the 'parish system' failed and the forging ahead of the institution gained momentum: on one hand was workhouse expansion, on the other, mental hospital development. The great revolution in hospital building was most evident in the industrialised urban areas of London, Lancashire, the Midlands and Yorkshire. For example, within a 40 mile radius of Manchester, some 10 large mental hospitals were built between 1800 and 1850.

Victorian custodians

Living and working conditions in Victorian Britain were inadequate for many citizens. Long working hours, bad housing, overcrowding and large families, produced stress which in turn contributed to the rising tide of mental illness. The main problem was one of accommodation. People suffering from mental illness were cared for in a variety of places, from locked rooms in private houses to cells in public institutions. Bethlem was the only public hospital caring for the mentally ill at the beginning of the eighteenth century. Hospitals built during the eighteenth century were small, and by 1840, Hanwell, with 100 beds, was the largest psychiatric hospital in England. The failure of hospital development produced a strain on overcrowded workhouses. Minutes from Strabane workhouse, Northern Ireland, 1842, mention the proposed change of the nursery into a women's day room and the provision of refractory cells for use when paupers were 'outrageous in their conduct'.

The Victorians responded to the need for more accommodation. Money was available from the County Asylum Act, 1808, which empowered Justices of the Peace to raise money for the building of mental hospitals through a county rate. This could be said to be the beginning of our present mental hospital system. The new institutions were larger and more skilfully constructed, with fine entrances and beautiful grounds. Over 80 psychiatric hospitals were built during the Victorian era and these new institutions were governed better too. Their large agricultural estates provided self-sufficiency as well as occupation for the patients, who were better provided for than they had been in the workhouses, which, up to now, had been the only resort of the great majority. As mental hospitals began to multiply from 1845–1860, pauper patients rose from 6500 to 17 500. At Tyrone and Fermanagh Psychiatric Hospital, opened in 1853, the first patients were 85 paupers transferred from Omagh Union Workhouse.

The expansion of mental hospitals prior to 1850 was too rapid to recruit suitable staff. Many difficulties were experienced but the greatest handicap was lack of training. During this period the staff practised a rigid routine and used coercive measures such as locked doors, padded cells, seclusion, deprivation and curtailment of freedom, in order to get the patients to behave as they wished.

Moral managers

Many nineteenth-century writers maintain that a person may be responsible for his mental illness, in that his condition is due to something he did, rather than something which happened to him. The idea of personal responsibilty for madness was developed, and the possibility of the patient controlling and preventing it was studied. Rev. Barlow in *Man's Power Over Himself* (1840), claims that diseases of the brain, however distressing, may and do, where the mind is cultivated, leave the individual capable of knowing right from wrong. Barlow's idea was to encourage self-help and individual control rather than external controls of custodial psychiatry. J. S. Mill had similar views on moral management. According to this school of thought, physical restraint, coercion and exile were to be replaced by a 'philosophy of self' which highlighted the dual nature of man and the power of the will to prevent insanity.

The earliest and best known account of moral management is by Samuel Tuke (in his description of the York Retreat, 1813, founded in 1792). The Retreat practised moral management in contrast to the repressive systems of other mental hospitals.

Legal involvement

Though the laws of Britain took a passing interest in the mentally ill, albeit a minor one, they did not show any active involvement until 1845, when the Lunatics Act made all establishments which housed the mentally ill (including prisons and workhouses) liable to inspection. This was an encouraging advance since the mentally ill had no legal protection.

Lunacy and Treatment Acts

There was a prevailing need to encourage admission of the mentally ill who would benefit from early treatment. The Lunacy Act 1890 insisted on a magistrate's order before a patient could be admitted to the mental institution, which meant that his illness was well advanced before he entered for treatment. This setback was prolonged due to staff shortages during the First World War and it was not until 1930, when the Mental Treatment Act allowed voluntary admission, that the way for progress was open.

National Health Service Act

The 1948 National Health Service Act provided much-needed extra revenue from Central Government for mental hospital budgets. The majority of mental hospitals used this extra money to improve the internal environment for the patient through renovation and redecoration. Another advantage of the NHS was that it brought doctors and nurses working in mental hospitals into the mainstream of medicine.

The 1959 Mental Health Act

The 1959 Act had two major provisions. First, it made it possible for any patient to be admitted informally to any hospital which could provide treatment for him. This was an important change because it made the system of admission for the mentally ill the same as that which had always existed for the physically ill. Secondly, it placed a new emphasis on the care of mental patients in the community, rather than in custody or in hospital. Local authorities were encouraged to provide hostels, clubs and other facilities which would make the concept of community care a reality.

The Mental Health Act 1983

This Act subsequently replaced the 1959 Act. It made some changes to the 1959 Principal Act and introduced new legislation, expanding on existing provisions (see Chapter 32).

Hospital plans and reorganisation

The Mental Health Acts made no attempt to forecast the proportion of mentally ill who would in future be treated in psychiatric departments of general hospitals or in the community. The Hospital Plan 1962 did however produce figures. The plan assured that by 1975 there would be a reduction of roughly 40 per cent in the provision of hospital beds for the mentally ill in England and Wales, resulting in a reduction of beds in mental hospitals with relatively more beds in psychiatric units in general hospitals. However, like many other assessments, particularly those based on projections, the estimate dismissed far too lightly the increasing proportion of the elderly in the population. Nevertheless, we see today more patients being discharged from psychiatric hospitals, and the concept of psychiatric units and community hostels is forging ahead. A more recent advance, the Government plans to reorganise the NHS, outlined in the 1980 Consulatative Document, *Patients First*, and the recommendations for district psychiatric management teams given in the Nodder Report (*Organisational and Management Problems of Mental Illness Hospitals*, HMSO, 1980), when implemented will further co-ordinate hospital and community services for the psychiatric patient.

Physical involvement

The 1930's saw the introduction of physical treatments for psychiatric conditions. These were based on the belief that by altering the physical environment of brain cells by varying techniques, changes could be produced in the patient's mental state.

The first method introduced was *Insulin Coma Therapy* to relieve schizophrenic symptoms. A high degree of medical and nursing care was required during treatment (which involved up to 60 comas) and this alone may have caused much of the improvement. Secondly, the *Pre-frontal Leucotomy* was introduced to help patients suffering from extreme tension and agitation to become more relaxed. The operation involved disconnecting the conducting fibres from the frontal lobe to the rest of the brain. Initially the treatment was used without sufficient discrimination. In *Pre-frontal Leucotomy in a Thousand Cases*, 1947, the Board of Control warned against over-enthusiastic resort to it. Now modified, the treatment is only used for selected patients but it still has its critics. The third treatment introduced in the 1930s was *Electroconvulsive therapy (ECT)*. The method used today differs from the original injection technique and is said to give relief to depressive patients as well as helping in the treatment of schizophrenia and other conditions.

Chemical involvement

Basically a physical treatment, chemotherapy has had such an impact on mental disorder that it warrants individual recognition. First used in the early 1950's, the use of chemical preparations has completely changed the treatment and prognosis of many mental disorders. Their credit lies in their ability to reduce signs and symptoms, thus enabling more people to be treated in the community, in addition to making the hospitalised patient more amenable to recovery and early discharge. On the debit side they may produce side effects and are open to misuse.

Post war views

Since the introduction of the National Health Service in 1948, comments have been made which are resulting in more vigorous attempts to reduce the undesirable aspects of institutional care. Foremost amongst the critics is Dr. Russell Barton, who, in his book *Institutional Neurosis* (1959), suggests that the psychiatric hospitals of the preceding decades were responsible for chronic psychological illness in their patients because they cared for them so completely, thus rendering them incapable of and uninterested in caring for themselves. Erving Goffman, in *Asylums* (1960), refers to the psychiatric hospital as a total institution which houses large numbers in an enclosed environment cut off from society. He comments on the formal administration and control of communication by the staff, in a system which fails to recognise the patient as an individual.

Attempts to minimise the undesirable factors mentioned were evident in the work of Maxwell Jones who, in 1947, organised a therapeutic community at Henderson Hospital, Surrey.

Anti-psychiatry views

Within psychiatry there are contemporary critics who condemn some of the practices and theories on psychiatry and suggest alternative solutions to the problems of mental illness.

T. S. Szasz is the author of many books including *The Myth of Mental Illness* (1976), *The Manufacture of Madness* (1973) and *The Age of Madness* (1975). He is a professor of psychiatry and a practising psychiatrist in New York who believes that it is false and immoral for society (i.e. government, legislature, hospitals, psychiatrists etc.) to view the mentally ill person as being psychologically and socially inferior to those not afflicted. This view enables society to intervene and care for the mental patient on the grounds that he is incapable and cannot choose for himself.

According to Szasz, this view removes personal responsibility from the mentally ill person and permits society to inflict treatments and incarcerate the sufferer in an institution, often against his will, on the basis that it is in the patient's best interest to do so.

R. D. Laing is the author of books such as *The Divided Self* (1970) and *Sanity, Madness and the Family* (with A. Esterson, 1970), which have a wide readership appeal among the general public, especially the younger generation. Laing is a practising psychiatrist who takes the view that schizophrenia is not really an illness and schizophrenics are not sick as such, but rather it is society which is sick and uses the schizophrenic as its scapegoat. Schizophrenia is not a disease in one person, but a crazy way in which the whole group functions. It is not a disease process of *soma* or *psyche* cause but a 'microsocial crisis situation' in which one member of the group (usually a family group) is elected by process to become the patient.

H. J. Eysenck is an advocate of the division of psychiatry into two independent parts: one organic and one behavioural. He argues in his publication *The Future of Psychiatry* (1975) that disorders such as schizophrenia and manic depressive psychosis are organic and should be treated by medically trained psychiatrists, while neurotic disorders should be treated by psychologists.

The psychiatric hospital today

Despite the progression to community care, half the hospital beds in Britain today are psychiatric. (It is necessary to point out however that many of these are occupied by psychogeriatric patients.) Nevertheless, in our overcrowded psychiatric hospitals there is a rich variety of experiment. Some run day hospitals which

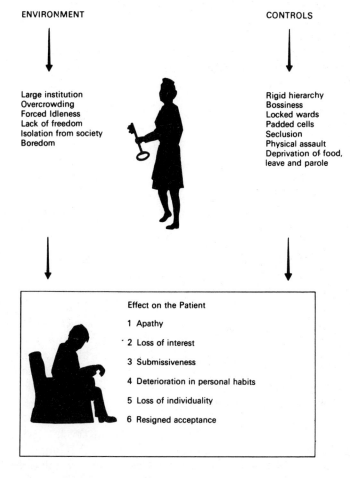

ENVIRONMENT

Large institution
Overcrowding
Forced Idleness
Lack of freedom
Isolation from society
Boredom

CONTROLS

Rigid hierarchy
Bossiness
Locked wards
Padded cells
Seclusion
Physical assault
Deprivation of food,
leave and parole

Effect on the Patient

1 Apathy

2 Loss of interest

3 Submissiveness

4 Deterioration in personal habits

5 Loss of individuality

6 Resigned acceptance

Fig. 1.2   Custodial practices (pre-1950)

provide both care and out-patient treatment. Other hospitals run their own hostels where patients can relearn independence prior to resettlement in the community.

Internally, psychiatric hospitals discourage the use of locked wards and the open door principle is extended to welcome the public in, as well as to let the patient out. Most wards have an integrated nursing staff and there is more activity now than ever existed in the custodial institution. It is difficult to think of an occupational or recreational activity which is not provided somewhere and there are numerous voluntary agents participating in the hospital services. Most psychiatric hospitals boast progressive industrial therapy units which are linked to local industry. Many more provide specialist units for treating adolescent problems and alcohol and drug dependent patients.

In conclusion, the modern psychiatric hospital is more dynamic than at any time in its history, despite the many obstacles evident, and there is a new drive to interact more with the society which it serves.

2

Hospitalisation and the Patient

The hospital as an organisation

The majority of people spend a large proportion of their professional life and leisure time in various organisations such as schools, clubs and associations. Most organisations need contributions from their members: a club may ask a fee for the use of its amenities, and the hospital that employs nurses to work for the achievement of their goals expects on its part to be able to exert control over those nurses, because control is implicit in an organisation. Controls are necessary and exist for the achievement of the hospital's goals which are to provide care and treatment for members of the public.

To ensure the public obtain the best care and treatment, the hospital uses many resources and must employ more and more people. In addition to the team of doctors and nurses, there are social workers, psychologists, occupational therapists, physiotherapists, domestic staff and so on. This collection of people requires to be organised and nature's characteristic organisation tends to a ranked system in which each person has a place: those above him to whom he is responsible, and those below who are responsible to him.

The organisation of hospital staff may appear strange and bewildering to the patient and his family. Rules, regulations and routines are a necessary evil for the smooth running of the service, but sometimes they make organisations look inhuman. For this reason, efforts are made to consider the individual and promote good communications for the benefit of the patient and his family.

The effects of hospitalisation on the patient

When patients are admitted to hospital they enter a strange new world. Meals are at a set time, there are new faces to get used to, there is communal sharing with reduced privacy and so on. The family link is broken and the patient must now learn to share with others. The patient's reaction to his new situation may include the following:

Anxiety

Quite naturally, patients are anxious when hospitalised. They have worries such as 'Who is going to look after my family?' and 'Will I lose my job?' These thoughts can be a constant source of anxiety which may delay recovery. Some patients may have numerous vague worries of an unsure nature, while others, once settled, may attach their anxiety to something specific such as the treatment they are receiving.

Regression and dependence

All human beings have the capacity to regress to an earlier stage of development and the hospital environment may be favourable to this process.

Not since infancy will the patient have been so nourished and tended or have been so dependent on others. The more helpless the patient's illness makes him, the more dependent he may become. Additionally, the nature of his illness may be such that he is looking for a place in which he can hide away and feel secure. Consequently, it is very important for the hospital staff to balance the patient's need for dependence and security against the therapeutic aims which are to promote independence and self-help.

Independence

Some patients may dislike hospital dependency and fight it, sometimes to their disadvantage. They may refuse treatment and nursing care by asking for their discharge long before they are ready for it. Also, some patients may feel they are a burden on the hospital and may struggle to help themselves rather than ask the nursing staff. This may apply particularly to elderly patients who tend to resist dependence. On the other hand, it is important for the nurse to appreciate that some patients may be too shy or embarrassed to ask for help with intimate problems.

Withdrawal

Mental illness may cause some patients to become self-absorbed and preoccupied with body sensations and personal problems. Matters are not helped by hospitalisation whereby the patient is separated from his home with its familiar values, routines, friends and relatives. Loss of contact with the outside world may limit his thinking to the immediate ward environment and his role as a sick person.

The sheltered hospital environment may make the patient become remote from ordinary events to the extent that he loses the confidence to resume normal life again. Consequently, steps must be taken from the time of the patient's admission to encourage contact with doctors, nurses, social workers and other patients, and to keep up contacts with relatives and friends.

Frustration and boredom

A day in hospital can be long and tedious for many patients. After a period, the routine can become predictable to the point of monotony: the endless round of getting up, taking pills, seeing the doctor and eating meals. Hospitals can be very frustrating for patients if adequate communication outlets are not provided to enable them to air their points of view and queries. These factors are not helped by the communal aspect of ward life whereby the patient must wait his turn to see the doctor or nurse.

The patient arrives in hospital

The attitudes of patients arriving in hospital vary considerably Most enter informally with anticipation of what lies ahead but hopeful of recovery. Others enter formally, often against their wishes, and may show resentment, resistance, and refusal to co-operate. Relatives may show concern and may not fully understand the patient's illness and its prognosis. The nurse will find the patient and relatives in great need of reassurance and should always aim to provide this during the admission procedure. There are three important areas to be considered when thinking about admissions:

The reception

Objectives

(1) To establish rapport with patients and relatives.
(2) To reassure and orientate.

The nurse should approach the situation in a pleasant and friendly manner. She should introduce herself and address the patient and his relatives individually. The patient should not be rushed but allowed time to orientate himself to his new circumstances. The nurse should adopt an interest in him and show warmth and sympathy for his feelings. The relatives should be guided to a quiet room and put at ease with a cup of tea. Their queries should be dealt with and someone left to talk with them while the patient is being settled in.

The admission

Objectives

(1) To attend to documentation and possessions.
(2) To inform the doctor of the patient's arrival.
(3) To prepare the patient for the physical examination.
(4) To observe the patient's physical and mental state.
(5) To involve two nurses in checking and recording valuables.
(6) To enlist the relatives' help when checking and recording admission data from confused and uncooperative patients.

When the patient is settled and at ease, the nurse should complete the admission forms, check and record valuables, examine and record property and obtain medicines and tablets for the doctor's attention. Ward rules should be adhered to regarding the amount of money the patient can retain and whether scissors, razor blades and matches are to be removed.

During the procedure the nurse should be discreetly observing the patient with a view to making a report on his general condition in the nurse's notes. She should observe the patient's attitude to hospitalisation, his appearance, behaviour, conversation, physical state, mental symptoms, temperature, pulse and respiration (TPR), height and weight. A urine sample should also be taken and tested.

Introduction to the ward

Objectives

(1) To introduce the patient to the ward, fellow patients, and staff.
(2) To follow the doctor's instructions on treatment.
(3) To protect the patient from the initial stresses of the ward.
(4) To protect the therapeutic environment of the ward from the patient's symptoms should they be disruptive.

The nurse can further help the patient to feel welcome and secure by introducing him to ward patients and staff. The ward routine should be explained and a conducted tour to include location of offices, lounge, sleeping accommodation, toilets, dining room and bathroom is necessary. The nurse should be prepared to give the patient extra attention until he is settled and familiar with the ward and other patients.

Note on physical examination

The nurse must prepare the patient for a physical examination. The procedure may add to his insecurity and be a source of embarrassment. The nurse should explain that the examination is routine for all new patients. The patient should be given the opportunity to prepare himself with a bath and the nurse should ensure that the examination is private and reassuring.

Patient status

On entering hospital patients will have varying roles and status based on their culture, occupation and social class. Many will leave these behind but some may find it difficult and have different expectations from those of the hospital staff. From the nursing viewpoint all patients have equal but special status in that they are the most important people in the hospital. On the other hand, patients may not consider their status to be high because they are not always free to make decisions or to exercise responsibility for what happens to them, this being in the hands of the doctors and nurses.

The nurse must be aware of factors in patient status which may influence her attitude towards some patients. For example, informal patients are sometimes perceived as having a higher status than formal patients because they have more rights under the law, in terms of the right to voluntary discharge, the right to refuse treatment and the right to leave of absence. Occasionally, informal patients regard themselves as having higher status and an entitlement to more favours from the nursing staff than compulsory patients. The nurse must guard against this by showing that rules and routines are necessary in the interest of all.

Anxiety and admission

In her research project, *Patient Anxiety on Admission to Hospital* (1975), Barbara Franklin states, 'an important part of the nurse's function involves relieving the anxiety of patients when they are admitted on the ward'. She goes on to say that the nurse must be able to recognise the symptoms of anxiety, and know the technique to employ for relieving it in just the same way as she must know how to cope with pain or other physical symptoms. (See Recommended Reading List.)

Recognising Anxiety

Anxiety can relate to any situation or illness and may show itself in the patient's behaviour by a variety of ways, such as:
- Increased talking; blocking of speech; restlessness, dry mouth; lump in throat sensation
- Profuse sweating; palpitations, pallor, fainting; tremors
- Diarrhoea; abdominal 'fullness', nausea and vomiting; rapid breathing; rapid pulse
- Fatigue; frequency of micturition; loss of appetite; insomnia; headaches

In severe cases the patient may be immobilised in thought and action and may experience a feeling of panic or terror – temporary personality disintegration may occur. Signs and symptoms of anxiety are usually evident during the physical examination and nursing assessment. The nursing assessment should include checking TPR, blood pressure (B/P) and urine analysis.

Preventing anxiety

Anxiety is such a commonplace symptom that it would be difficult to prevent its occurrence. Nevertheless, hospital staff can do much to minimise it.

1 Humanising the hospital

Bureaucratic factors such as red tape, petty restrictions and rules for the sake of rules should be kept to a minimum. The emphasis should be on personality rather than impersonality. All staff must be friendly and understanding, they must show a willing concern to help and at all times appear approachable. They should be aware of anxiety-producing factors and make an effort to present them in a way which will not lead to tension or fear. Staff should not deliberately avoid patients who need constant reassurance and neither should they be secretive or project attitudes which may provoke anxiety.

2 Maintaining a stress-free ward environment

It is up to the ward team to create a relaxing ward environment. Care must be taken to avoid aspects of management and

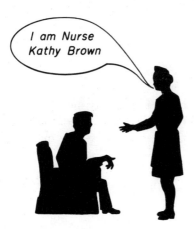

Personality rather than impersonality   **Fig. 2.1** Preventing anxiety

interpersonal relationships which produce strains and tensions. Friction between staff members may result in uneasiness in the ward atmosphere and be a source of anxiety to some patients. Good communications between staff and patients are important and opportunities should be created to allow patients to verbalise anxieties they may have regarding routines, procedures and treatments.

3 Early mobilisation of team members

Anxiety among patients can be prevented by prompt introduction to the team member who is best able to give advice and help. For example, patients concerned about financial problems or occupation should be seen early on by the social worker, while those concerned about medical treatment can be reassured by a friendly explanatory talk from the doctor or nurse.

Time is needed when helping the anxious patient and though reassurance maybe difficult and unrewarding, it is necessary.

Fig. 2.2 Relieving anxiety

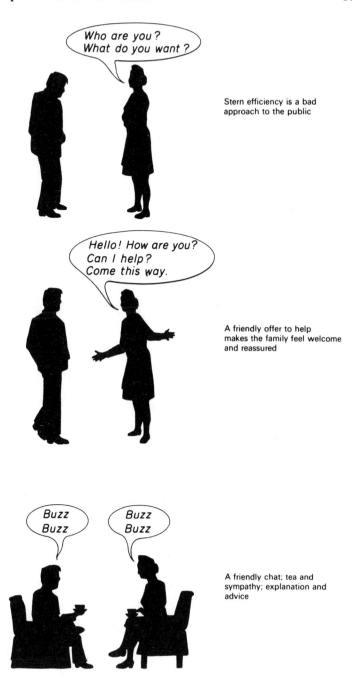

Fig. 2.3 Reducing the effects of hospitalisation on relatives

Relieving anxiety

Some general nursing points

The nurse should:

(1) Be friendly and give the patient her name and introduce him to other staff and patients. She should explain ward routines and encourage him to keep familiar objects, items of clothing etc.

(2) Explain to the patient that his stay in hospital will be as short as possible and the best way to help himself and his family is to settle and get well quickly.

(3) Ensure that staff are always available to discuss his problems and if he is worrying about something or someone at home, reassure him that those problems are being attended to. Listen and answer questions tactfully.

(4) Promote confidence and ease insecurity and uncertainty.

(5) Respect privacy and avoid embarrassing the patient.

(6) Explain procedures and treatments.

(7) Attempt to divert the patient's mind from his worries by changing the topic.

(8) Never tell the patient to pull himself together.

(9) Avoid panic and uncertainty herself as this may provoke further anxiety in the patient.

(10) If necessary, stay with the patient, as her presence and closeness will do more to soothe him than anything else.

3
Ward Organisation

'Therapeutic community' is the term commonly used to describe definite organisational features employed in the management of psychiatric patients which are considered to be beneficial to patient recovery.

Aims of the therapeutic community

(1) To promote closer relationships between staff and patients by encouraging a flexible ward organisation which is open to change, according to the individual and collective needs of the patients.
(2) To mobilise the interests, skills and enthusiasm of patients and staff through freedom of action, respectively to create their own optimal treatment and social environment and to try to understand anti-social behaviour from the patient.
(3) To motivate patients by allowing them an active and rewarding role in the care and treatment programmes which take cognisance of their problems.
(4) To encourage mutual discussion of problems, anxieties, resentments and frustrations by creating free and open communication.

Therapeutic organisation

Though the ultimate aim is to develop the hospital as a therapeutic unit, it is on the ward where therapeutic practice is most important. It is here that the patient spends most of his time, makes his contacts and receives his treatment.

Ward organisation should convey a healing message to each patient which will promote thoughts such as: 'This is a good place and I know I can get well here', rather than an untherapeutic one which is more likely to promote thoughts such as 'I've made a mistake by coming here' or 'This place will make me worse'.

The importance of the ward in the recovery process merits a closer consideration of the features which are conducive to a therapeutic environment. These will be discussed under two main headings, the first covering the static organisation (which includes staff structure and physical arrangement) and the second dealing with the dynamic organisation (which includes ward objectives and functioning in terms of communication, staff/patient interaction and organised activities).

Static aspects

Staff structure

Ward staff are the immediate treatment personnel (nurses, doctor, occupational therapists etc.), and the supportive servicing personnel are cleaners, caterers and those responsible for maintainance. The nursing staff occupy a permanent existence on the ward, providing a 24 hour presence, and other ward personnel visit the ward as clients dictate. Nursing staff are organised in a hierarchical structure and coexist with other personnel as illustrated in the diagram below.

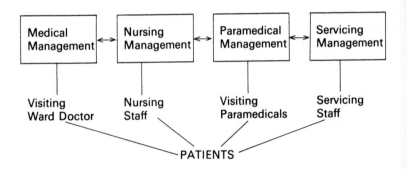

Ward arrangement

Wards should be spacious and arranged to promote comfort and relaxation. Decor should be tasteful with furniture arranged for the patient's needs and comfort. Each ward must have adequate storage facilities for each individual's possessions. Toilet and washing facilities should be private and the ward should be clean, well lit and adequately ventilated.

Ward routine

The main routine landmarks are usually static to ensure the smooth functioning of the ward. This is necessary in the general interest of all patients. Most wards arrange a skeleton routine based on meal times, with varying degrees of flexibility in the inbetween periods.

For example, the recovering schizophrenic patient should be introduced to a flexible routine to promote independence, while a geriatric patient may require a fairly rigid routine to ease confusion and allow for the slowing of his activity.

Dynamic aspects

Ward objectives

1 **Atmosphere.** The wards must foster an atmosphere of acceptance and understanding of anti-social behaviour rather than attempting to deal with it by arbitrary authority, restraint or sedation. It is important for nurses to ask 'What does this behaviour mean?' rather than 'What can we do to stop it quickly?'

2 **Learning.** The ward should encourage patients to learn how they can help each other and permit them to do so whenever possible. Staff must learn to share therapy skills with each other to gain a greater understanding of the meaning of personal relationships and a better capacity to use them.

3 **Development.** The ward staff, ward resources and activities must be arranged to promote the development of the patient to become independent and to make his own decisions to the maximum degree that his illness will permit.

4 **Communications.** Communications should be free and open. Opportunities should be created by organising ward life in such a way that both staff and patients have the maximum time to exchange freely their views, criticisms and feelings on matters which are important to them. This enables the creative contributions of patients and junior staff to be incorporated into the community. It follows that those in postions of authority, in all grades of staff, must be able to accèpt suggestions and criticism without making their juniors feel out on a limb.

Ward communications can be promoted through various channels:

Patient/staff ward meetings

These should be held at least once weekly and should include the ward doctor, nurses, patients, a domestic representative and paramedicals. Such meetings are crucial for communication, development and learning.

Usually no particular subject is chosen but generally the topics which emerge include grumbles about routine, food, ward incidents, treatment, ward and hospital activities, staff relationships and personal problems. All staff involved in the ward should make a special effort to be there. If staff show good interest it encourages patients to attend.

Staff meetings

A weekly staff meeting helps promote successful ward functioning. Staff meetings should be an informal part of the ward routine so that all staff can be free to attend. Failure to include the staff meeting as a part of the ward routine often results in a falling off in staff attendance and loss of continuity in discussion.

Ward staff meetings

- Provide an outlet for staff to discuss their views, criticisms, suggestions, problems, anxieties and opinions
- Enable team members to discuss and evaluate treatment and nursing strategy
- Help staff to share each others' problem areas and understand their roles
- Discuss feedback from patients' meetings
- Provide a learning situation for junior staff
- Promote therapeutic relationships and add impetus to staff morale and job satisfaction

Psychodrama

The ward should create opportunities for patients to be actively involved in their own recovery. Instead of talking about their problems psychodrama groups encourage patients to act out situations involving conflict with the help of the nurse and the rest of the group. Situations can be chosen from the patient's own life experience from the past, present or imagined future. Scenes are enacted in the 'here-and-now' and other group members play supporting roles in the protagonist's life drama. This exploration of the truth through drama involves an extension of everyday life experience. It makes use of man's ability to be spontaneous in making his life as he wants it to be. In psychodrama the patient can experiment with his life without being ridiculed or punished for his mistakes.

Staff functioning

It is generally accepted that the psychiatric patient benefits from cohesiveness of the various staff members involved in his care and treatment. For this purpose a team approach is used. The psychiatric team consists of staff members who have a specialised role to play. These roles may overlap to some extent and this may produce friction and conflict. Such disturbance can be minimised however, if roles are clearly understood and participants are free to discuss difficulties as they arise.

The team's success depends on close collaboration between members with freedom to use their professional skills and understanding with the patient in an atmosphere of mutual respect. If the working environment fails to allow for members to express themselves, the patient loses a professional service that is rightfully due to him.

It is important for the team to recognise that its members may, at times, need the support and understanding help of others in stressful situations. The group work of the team implies that each member should focus his interest on the patient and share his observations, skills and knowledge with the other members so that no one feels he is working alone with the patient.

Sometimes increased continuity of patient contact is encouraged through 'primary nursing' whereby each patient is allocated to a particular nurse in the staff team for all his basic support. This nurse becomes his personal counsellor, teacher and friend.

THE CARING TEAM

Immediate team members	Supporting members
Psychiatrist	Voluntary services officer
Psychiatric nurse	Pharmacists
Occupational therapist	Technicians
Recreational therapist	Hospital administrator
Remedial gymnast	Beauticians
Psychologist	Chaplin
Psychiatric social worker	Resettlement officer
Industrial therapy officer	Maintenance supervisor
	Tailor, dressmaker etc.

Community team contacts

Social workers	General practitioner
Voluntary agencies	Patient associations
Hostel supervisors	Mental health associations
Community services	Family and relatives

Other factors promoting ward dynamism include:

Open doors

The idea that psychiatric ward doors can be open to allow patients more freedom is now widely accepted and practised by most hospitals. The open ward benefits both staff and patients. Tensions are reduced, violence declines and escapes are no longer a problem. The nursing staff are free from the over-protective, mistrustful task of counting patients in at the door and escorting them each time they leave the ward. This allows the staff to develop more meaningful relationships based on trust and enables them to give more attention to therapy rather than custody.

Though the wandering patient can be a problem, this should not be allowed to lead to curtailment of all the ward patients' freedom. The open ward encourages the patient to retain his dignity and self-respect which is essential in giving him the confidence he needs for recovery.

Mixed sexes

Encouragement is given for contact between the sexes at all levels in the therapeutic community. Male and female patients mix together in work therapy and recreational activities. Also, male and female patients are sometimes nursed on the same ward staffed by male and female nurses.

Mixed wards are considered to be more therapeutic in that they help correct anti-social behaviour, promote interaction between patients and staff, and encourage patients to improve their personal hygiene and appearance. Nurses must ensure patient privacy on mixed wards and respect the views of those who may not be happy in such an environment.

Work therapy

Hospitalisation which includes enforced idleness leads to boredom, preoccupation, loss of self-respect, withdrawal and anti-social behaviour. One of the main aims of work therapy, therefore, is to prevent regression and to stimulate the patient's interest in activities which are therapeutic in the short term and rewarding in the long term and which will help the patient acquire skills which will facilitate his return to work when he leaves hospital.

1 Occupational therapy. This therapy is usually carried out in either a special building set aside for the purpose or on the ward where the patient resides. The choice of location for activities will vary with the particular needs of the patient. Skilled occupational therapists and nursing staff work together in conducting the therapy. Its purpose is to help to lessen symptoms, relieve boredom, improve concentration, build confidence, sharpen memory, improve relationships, provide outlets for energy and opportunities to evaluate the patient's performance.

2 Industrial therapy. Industrial therapy units are now well established in most psychiatric hospitals. The aim of this activity differs somewhat from occupational therapy in that it is not far away from a normal work situation. The unit is organised on factory lines where the patient can learn to keep time, care for tools, accept work discipline and participate in union activities. The type of work available is graded so that patients can progress from one grade to another and can derive pleasure, improve concentration and receive financial reward, which promotes a sense of independence.

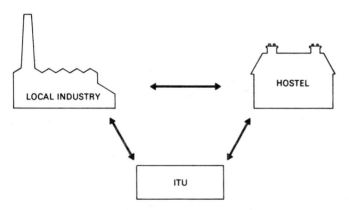

Local factories supply the industrial therapy unit
with components for assembly. When the patient is
a proficient worker he may leave hospital and
live in a hostel or flat

Fig. 3.1 Industrial therapy

In this activity the industrial therapy officer becomes works manager, personnel officer, salesman and clerk rolled into one. It is his responsibility to gain co-operation from local industry to supply his unit with a variety of occupations and to assess each patient so that he is placed in a task suitable to his needs and level of rehabilitation. In some instances hospitals accept patients on their staff and have found the arrangement satisfactory. Some convalescent patients have been able to commence paid employment in local industry and remain living in the hospital until they find accommodation in a flat or hostel.

The nurse's role in work therapy

No patient in the hospital should be excluded from work therapy and it is the duty of the nurse to ensure that each patient's needs are met. The nurse's role develops by working with the patient in practical situations. She should be given an opportunity to form a closer relationship through which encouragement can be given. The therapy also enables the patient to become more involved in his own rehabilitation thus encouraging independence and self help in the recovery process. It is important for the nurse to encourage patients to attend the therapy departments and to be inventive in providing occupational activities for those who are unable to leave the ward.

Recreational therapy

The provision of a considerable amount of recreational activity is an important aspect of the therapeutic community. Such recreational activities are a natural and necessary part of a favourable hospital environment, and are therapeutic in so far as they contribute to the recovery process. This therapy promotes relaxation, confidence, interaction and the development of social skills, and prevents boredom, apathy and frustration. It also relieves tension, provides outlets for expressing social drives and gives opportunities for patients to plan and organise for themselves.

Types of activity. The patient is given access to such items as daily newspapers, library books, popular magazines, radio, television and a piano, as well as facilities for various games such as dominoes, chess, cards, darts and table tennis.

Recreational programmes. A good recreational programme offers a graded series of experiences. At one extreme would be the passive role of spectator at a game, whereby the patient may obtain release of tension by identification with the active competitors. At the other extreme would be a highly competitive role such as playing a vigorous game of cricket or tennis. All types of interests can be accommodated in the programme and opportunities afforded for competitive, educational, cultural, expressive, social and intellectual experiences.

The programme of activities should be flexible to allow for individualism and, when preparing the programme, the team must encourage the patients to become involved in planning their own activities either on an individual or group basis.

The recreational therapist

Recreational therapy is concerned with helping patients to express themselves through various social group activities. A qualified therapist usually works with groups in a wide range of activities in which she has achieved a degree of competence. She may take the leadership in planning parties, social clubs, group outings, educational programmes, cinema shows and various other activities.

Occupational therapy

Assessment	*Variety in activities*	*Feedback*
Patient's illness	Basket making	Therapist's reports
Treatment	Rug making	Team meetings
Age	Pottery	Nurses' reports
Intelligence	Painting	Patient/staff meetings
Physical handicaps	Needlework	
Length of stay	Beauty care	
Previous occupation	Domestic activities	
	Woodwork	
	Assembly	
	Gardening	

4
Psychiatric Nursing
Skills and Duties

The psychiatric nurse must possess a variety of skills which may be seen as follows:

Caring skills

These skills are necessary for the physical well-being of the patient. They include such acts as feeding, bathing, dressing, administering treatments, observing, comforting and generally maintaining physical health. They also involve caring for psychiatric patients who are physically ill or helpless and thus require things to be done for them.

Therapy skills

A significant part of the nurse's time will involve the use of therapy skills in both individual and group situations, as a means of promoting recovery. The nurse must participate with her patients in their daily activities and use resourcefulness when planning care in order to promote interaction, motivation, learning experiences and rehabilitation. She must give support to her patients and encourage them to have confidence in their ability to overcome their problems.

Communications skills

Patients may communicate by various forms of behaviour both consciously and unconsciously. For example, they may transmit attitudes, thoughts and feelings using the spoken or written word, body movements and physical signals, or by expression through paintings, drawings and so on. In addition to interpreting communication modes the nurse must also learn to communicate successfully with patients, their relatives and her team colleagues.

Administrative skills

These include skills in basic management such as planning and executing nursing and rehabilitation programmes and organising other therapeutic activities. They also include requisitioning ward supplies, keeping records, maintaining charts, organising patient groups, recording minutes and writing reports.

Counselling skills

Counselling skills are concerned with the art of talking, listening, and encouraging discussion for the purpose of helping patients to recognise their problems and to assist them in finding solutions.

Protective skills

Some patients may attempt to inflict self-injury during the acute stage of their illness. Others, especially confused patients, may wander and come to harm. It is the duty of the nurse to protect such patients until their recovery reduces any risk of injury or accident.

Socialising skills

Socialising skills are concerned with the nurse's ability to discard her authoritative role and share social and recreational activities with her patients, such as playing games, visiting local amenities, dancing, party-going, etc. Though the nurse may discard her more strict regimes (including her uniform) she continues to act as an agent for the patient to learn the rules expected for social intercourse. The patient benefits by becoming more relaxed and freer in interpersonal relationships, thus gaining confidence to function in the social setting. (See also Social skills, pp. 32–33.)

Technical skills

Part of the treatment may require the use of machines or other technical apparatus. It is necessary for the nurse to be skilled in the procedures for the preparation, use and maintenance of the equipment used. In all procedures the nurse must put emphasis on technical skills, patient comfort and safety.

Public relations skills

Health Service consumers are members of the public. Whether the consumer is ill in bed, visiting loved ones, enquiring by phone or seeking information, it is important for the nurse to be articulate and relaxed so she can deal with the consumer in a reassuring and helpful manner without causing frustration or alarm in the process. It involves skills in talking, listening, anticipating, understanding, caring and, above all, in having patience and showing interest in the problems of others.

Observation skills

The nurse will learn to become a skilled observer of her patients, knowing their individual reactions and their reactions within the group. Slight variations in a patient's appearance and behaviour may be very significant to the experienced nurse. Some psychiatric patients may be uncommunicative and unable to complain if they are feeling unwell. In such circumstances the nurse is the eyes and ears for the patient through her function as a skilled observer.

Professional skills

The nurse is a member of a profession and both her profession and the public will have expectations which apply not only to her work situation but also to her role as a citizen. The nurse will learn to develop a professional character and dignity which will enable her to balance these roles in a way that will neither disappoint nor frustrate these expectations. The nurse is also bound to a professional code of ethics which expects loyalty to colleagues and a concern for patient confidentiality.

The community psychiatric nurse

The current approach is very much to recognise the desirability of treating the mentally ill patient in his own home or other community accommodation. The nurse is an integral part of community care services which include protective care and after-care for those who require encouragement and support to become fully integrated into the community.

The nurse will be a member of a team (some hospital based, some community based) whose primary objective is the return of the in-patient to a normal happy life in the community. To care for the patient at home boosts his self-esteem and removes him from the dependence of hospitalised care. The community care team includes nurses, health visitors, voluntary workers, district nurses, family doctors and social workers.

The community nurse's role

The nurse may be hospital based in a community nurses' department and travel to her clients each day, or she may operate from a health centre or a nurses' out-patient clinic. Her duties will include:

1 *Returning hospitalised patients to the community*

(1) Establishing a relationship with the patient prior to discharge and making contact with the family in order to understand the home conditions and prepare the family for the patient's return.

(2) Obtaining alternative accommodation if the patient has no relatives or family links are poor, and establishing his relationships with community team members.

(3) Obtaining personal services when needed (e.g. attendance allowance, sickness benefit).

(4) Advising ward staff on the education of the patient for his new role and educating the community on the problems of the mentally ill.

2 *Maintaining long-term patients in the community*

(1) Visiting the home of the patient and noting the patient's progress.

(2) Reporting to the doctor in charge and to the responsible nursing officer. (The nurse may report to the patient's family doctor in the first instance.)

(3) Observing that medication, other treatments and medical appointments are continued as ordered by the doctor, and consulting with the doctor should any change in treatment be indicated.

(4) Observing and dealing with side effects of medication.

(5) Working in conjunction with the social worker and disablement resettlement officer to obtain employment for the patient.

The community psychiatric nurse's role may bring her into contact with the following care agencies: psychiatric units in general hospitals, hostels and other half-way accommodation; supervised lodgings and boarding out schemes; sheltered workshops and factories; day centres; social clubs and ex-patient clubs; child guidance clinics; voluntary organisations; social service departments and housing departments.

Increasingly the community psychiatric nurse is playing a role in the early recognition of mental illness and prevention through counselling, family therapy and crisis intervention.

Summary of the psychiatric nurse's general duties

The nurse's skills will be operative within her overall role and duties which may be summarised as follows:
- Establishing relationships with patients and staff
- Observing and supervising patients
- Feeding, washing, dressing, reassuring and supporting patients and sharing activities such as playing games, occupations, discussion groups and so on
- Explaining routines and administering treatments
- Listening and talking to patients, showing courtesy to relatives
- Maintaining the patients' general health by giving attention to ward cleanliness; heating, lighting and ventilation of wards; serving of meals; clothing of patients; exercise, rest and sleep and the prevention of accidents and infection
- Requisitioning ward supplies and caring for equipment
- Practising good economy of ward resources
- Implementing nursing care and rehabilitation programmes
- Evaluating care

Allocation to a new ward

On her allocation to a new ward the nurse will be introduced to the ward team, its objectives and function.

General objectives. The mental and physical well-being of patients and the harmonious function of ward staff.

Specific objectives. These will vary and depend on the type of ward, e.g.:

(a) *Acute wards*. Here, the immediate aim will be to protect the patient from the effects of his acute symptoms and begin his recovery with a view to an early return to society.

(b) *Long-term wards* will put the emphasis on consolidating the patients's recovery and progressing with rehabilitation towards a way of life which is orientated towards normality and self-help and eventual return to the outside community.

Note on social skills

Many 'psychiatric nursing skills' are interchangeable with social skills. Social skills are components of social interaction and are described in the next two chapters.

The social skills model conceptualises man as pursuing social and other goals, acting according to rules, monitoring his performance in the light of continuous feedback from his environment (Trower, 1978). Argyle (1967) considered features in social skills as:

1 Establishing rapport with the other person.
2 Keeping the person in play.
3 Motivating the client.
4 Reducing anxiety.
5 Concern of the performer with the impression they are making on others.

Social Competence

Argyle identified the components of social competence as (1) perceptual sensitivity, (2) warmth and rapport, (3) repertoire of social techniques, (4) flexibility, (5) energy, and (6) smooth response patterns.

Psychiatric nurses need to possess social skills for their function and also for patient rehabilitation because as Trower (1978) states 'some forms of mental disorder are caused or exacerbated by lack of social competence and can be cured or alleviated by means of training in social skills'. The two important skills are:

1 Communications. Communicative competence, as Bell (1976) describes communication, recognises verbal communications as a social skill as well as a linguistic skill. Ruesch (1967) suggested that there were four characteristics in successful communications. These are:

(a) *Feedback.* This is the process of the receiver relaying back to the sender the effects of the communication.

(b) *Appropriateness.* The reply should be relevant and related to the initial message.

(c) *Efficiency.* A clear message with simple words and enough time for the receiver to take it in.

(d) *Flexibility.* Not authoritative or permissive.

2 Interpersonal Relationships. Paplav (1952) described the nurse patient relationship as the 'crux of psychiatric nursing'. It can be viewed as the core of all psychiatric nursing therapies (see Chapter 6).

Interpersonal techniques or *strategies* may be used widely by the nurse for dealing with a variety of problems. A strategy should be developed for each problem (e.g. dealing with aggressive people) and put into practice when the problem arises. The nurse should also make use of therapies for achieving strategies wherever possible. For example, behaviour therapy, psychodrama, psychotherapy and group therapy.

5
Developing
Nursing Skills

The following skills are important for successful patient care and as such will be discussed more fully here.

Talking

The art of conversation may be difficult for some and the nurse must learn to talk with patients about a variety of things (particularly those that will interest the patient). She should never ignore the patient and always take the opportunity to say 'Hello!' 'Good morning!' 'How are you?' and so on. She should talk to him about his job, interests, likes and dislikes, a news topic, or simply establish conversation and allow him to talk things over with her.

The nurse should avoid talking down to patients or using obscure or technical terminology. She should talk to them at their level and encourage them to clarify the meaning of their communication. She should be honest. She should always be interested in what they are saying but not go along with their delusions and hallucinations. She should always appear attentive and not pretend to understand what they are talking about when she does not. She should ask them to clarify a reference or say something like this: 'I don't quite follow you', or 'Let's go over it again'.

The nurse should not feel guilty about spending time talking with patients. It is part of her role. She should not moralise about something the patient may say because she finds it unacceptable to her own upbringing or sub-culture.

Sometimes nurses may begin to feel that there is no point in continuing to talk to uncommunicative patients because they never talk back. The inherent danger may be that the nurse will regard this patient's lack of communication as normal and stop talking to him.

Talking to elderly patients, patients with confusion and patients suffering from organic dementia presents additional problems. Such patients may be unable to follow a normal conversation; misunderstanding can occur more readily and hearing may be impaired. In these circumstances, the nurse should speak in a precise manner; she should use expressions and hand movements in support, speak loudly if necessary and be prepared to repeat herself until the patient grasps what she is saying.

Listening

It could be argued that most people want to talk but few are prepared to listen. On the other hand, one must accept that barriers exist when it comes to revealing problems to others. How frequently one hears the comment, 'It's not everyone you can talk to.' The patient may have a problem that he needs to talk out with someone. He may have had the problem on his mind for many months and need to verbalise it so that he feels relief or understands it better. It is important therefore for the nurse to create the right atmosphere and let the patient be aware that she is the kind of person who is prepared to listen.

The skilled nurse learns not to probe but rather to listen. She will develop the art of repeating the odd phrase to show the patient that she is still listening. She will not be impatient and inattentive. She will organise her listening time so that she does not have to clock watch, thus giving the patient the feeling that he is keeping her from more important duties or that he is being a nuisance. She will respect the patient's confidences and will only reveal these to the doctor if they are considered relevant to his condition and if he does not wish to tell the doctor himself.

The nurse will not feel flattered because the patient confides in her rather than in the doctor; she will seek advice on matters which are within the province of the doctor. She will be a sympathetic listener but she will avoid becoming emotionally involved in the patient's problems. She will hear many things from her patient which may shock her but she will not condemn them.

Reassurance

Reassurance is an attempt to help the patient to feel better, to make him less afraid, to dispel his doubts, to allay his anxieties, to relieve tension, to help him understand his symptoms and to come to terms with his treatment, to help him accept that all is not lost and generally promote his self-confidence.

When reassuring the patient, it is not simply a matter of telling him that he is in good hands and everything will be all right. The nurse must give explanations; she must show understanding and patience; she must give attention and remain calm and she must comfort and spend time with the patient.

Patients may be reassured in a number of ways in response to a variety of circumstances and situations. Some of these are listed below and will be related to specific situations in later chapters:

- Explaining services, treatments and symptoms
- Listening to problems, giving advice, support and encouragement
- Staying with the patient and anticipating needs
- Remaining calm and instilling confidence
- Touching, holding hands and comforting
- Taking the patient's mind off his problems through activities
- Introducing a third party who may be able to help

Counselling

Patients will frequently bring problems to and seek advice from the nurse. The nurse should encourage the patient to talk through his problem and together they can identify the difficult areas. Once the problem is located the nurse can give guidance but she must avoid solving the problem for him. The aim of the counsellor must be to encourage the patient to make his own decisions and find his own solutions. The nurse should not suggest a particular solution, for then if it fails, the patient will blame the nurse. Neither should the nurse undermine the doctor/patient relationship by offering advice or suggestions which are contrary to those given by the doctor. Lastly, the nurse's role as a counsellor may concern her with problems of a very personal nature, therefore, the strictest confidence must be observed.

Suggestion

The nurse can do much for the patient by using simple suggestion. For example, some patients may be unable to stop brooding on their problems, others cannot express themselves, and some may be unable to use their free time constructively. The nurse can create activities and situations which will make the patient susceptible to participation. More directly, she can suggest topics for group discussion and hint at possible activities. She can also influence the patient by her own personality and actions. However, some patients, such as hysterics, may be too suggestible, so it is important that the activities presented to them are desirable.

Persuasion

A great deal of coaxing and persuading is needed when nursing some psychiatric patients. It may be necessary to encourage a patient to eat his meals, take his medication, attend the therapy department, mix with other patients and so on. The nurse will have to give a logical explanation to the patient for performing the action she desires from him. She should be calm and persistent and temper insistence with gentleness.

Supervision

Too much supervision can be restrictive and over-protective. The nurse must learn to balance the need for supervision against the need for freedom and individuality. While the patient's illness and treatment will largely determine the level of supervision, the nurse should understand that some patients may be sensitive and embarrassed by close supervision while it may make others feel secure. The criteria for the level of supervision should include such questions as 'Is it necessary for the patient's well-being and recovery?'

Continuous supervision

Patients requiring close supervision may include those with acute mania, disturbed schizophrenia, suicidal tendencies, senility, confusion, stupor, deterioration, withdrawal, drug dependence, disturbance of consciousness, anorexia nervosa, epilepsy and pre- and post-ECT.

Periodic supervision

All patients should be supervised during periods such as meals, medication, bathing, work, dressing and washing to ensure that these activities are performed.

Observation

Skilled observation is essential because by this means we can learn much about the patient's physical and mental condition. Through observation the nurse will understand the patient's behaviour and also aid the doctor in assessment and diagnosis. The nurse must not go about with her eyes closed if she is to be a valuable member of the psychiatric team.

Why do we observe?

We need to know and understand the patient. We must discover the kind of person he is, his mental and physical state, his behaviour and reaction in the ward situation, his interests and the way he responds to treatment and rehabilitation.

When do we observe?

Though the nurse must be observant at all times, there are occasions which provide more opportunities than others:

On admission – the nurse should:

(1) Note the patient's reaction to hospitalisation, e.g. level of anxiety, indifference and co-operation.

(2) Observe the patient's psychiatric symptoms, e.g. delusions, hallucinations, orientation, mood, insight and conversation.

(3) Note the patient's physical state, e.g. height, weight, colour, mobility, balance, sight, hearing, deformities, temperature, pulse and respiration, skin, hair and body cleanliness.

While sleeping – note sleep rhythm, restlessness, insomnia and effect of night medication.

On getting up – note the patient's manner of dressing, appearance, grooming and attention to hygiene.

At medication time – ensure that the patient takes his medication and always look for possible side effects.

During meals – note appetite, table manners, reactions to the meal, likes and dislikes and food refusal.

During activities – note the patient's reaction to work, recreation and so on. Observe his interests, progress, interaction and punctuality.

During visiting hours – note the patient's reaction to his visitors and observe his behaviour during visits.

Pattern of elimination – note frequency of micturition, diarrhoea or constipation.

Reporting

Reports are necessary to convey observations to all team members involved in the care of the patient. Good reporting should be factual and not based on assumptions. Reports should be clear and meaningful; the use of clichés, hospital jargon and abbreviations should be avoided where possible. For reference purposes, reports should be titled, dated and signed by the recorder.

Reports may take a number of forms and are generally classified as follows:

1 Administrative reports

Day and night reports are usually written to provide the nursing administrator with a general picture of ward events and patient changes. They do not give a detailed account of each patient's progress but merely record staff on duty, bed state, admissions, discharges, deaths, major treatments and dramatic or unusual changes. Such reports are forwarded to the unit nursing officer.

2 Ward reports

A more detailed ward report (the nursing care plan) remains on the ward to provide more information for the ward staff. Each team member should read this on commencing a shift of duty. Such reports mention all the patients on the ward and should consider their mental state, physical state, treatments, special observations and nursing care.

An individual record of the patient's behaviour and progress may be kept by making use of the nurses' notes. They provide a continuous picture and are included as part of the patient's case notes.

3 Medical reports

All medical reports relating to the patient's illness, circumstances and treatment are recorded in the medical case notes. As much of the information is confidential between doctor and patient, proper ethical codes should be practised regarding their content, use and storage.

6
Nursing Relationships

Developing nurse/patient relationships

There is no magic formula for learning how to develop and maintain satisfying human relationships. The task is not made easier when one considers the many variants in human relationships and the need for the nurse to balance some type of general relationship with all the patients on the ward against a more specific relationship with one particular patient or group of patients.

When the nurse is introduced to a ward she will be expected to care for different types of patients, some of whom are withdrawn, some excited, some suicidal, some anxious and so on. At first the nurse may be impressed with the apparently normal behaviour of some patients yet distressed with the disturbed behaviour of others. Initially all the patients will be strangers to the nurse and vice versa. Nevertheless, from this mutual uncertainty, relationships will develop which will vary in quality, intensity, and frequency of interaction.

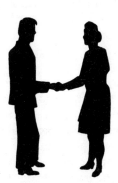

The nursing relationship is the core of the helping process

Fig. 6.1   The nursing relationship

Factors in relationship development

Initial contact and acceptance

First impressions are important and may influence the frequency of contact thereafter. Either the nurse or the patient may decide to discriminate in their relationships on the basis of the first contact and it is important for the nurse to be aware of this. From the nurse's viewpoint it is important that she accepts the patient and understands his behaviour. She should also be aware of aspects of her own personality such as attitudes and mannerisms, which may be off-putting to the patient.

Initially the nurse should be herself, use common sense, and act naturally and in a relaxed manner. She should show interest in her patients, accept each as an individual and allow for their differences. She should never talk down to her patients, make promises she cannot keep or break confidences without first consulting the patient. She should avoid giving the impression that the relationship is an attempt to psychoanalyse the patient and neither should she try too hard if the patient appears slow to relate to her.

Ignoring patients, talking down to them, breaking promises and trying too hard are all factors which may quickly 'switch off' a relationship.

Trust

Without a basis for trust it is difficult to form a therapeutic relationship between the nurse and her patient. Failure by the nurse to trust the patient may lead him to the conclusion that she is unhelpful and cannot be depended upon.

The patient may need time before he learns to trust the nurse; he may often bring with him a sense of mistrust based on experience. On the other hand, his mistrust may be due to his illness whereby he wrongly believes that the world is hostile and will ridicule or betray his secrets.

On occasions when the patient is unable to control his behaviour, the nurse must protect him where necessary but trust him to be able to cope eventually. At times she may have physically to prevent the patient from dangerous acts and show disapproval towards certain behaviours, but the fact that she continues to place trust in the relationship may prove to him that he is acceptable even though his behaviour is not.

Emotional involvement

The extent to which the nurse should allow herself to become emotionally involved with the patient is open to debate. One could put forward the view that her relationship is strictly a professional one and requires that she should not identify too closely with the patient or become emotionally over-involved or over-concerned with his personal problems. The inherent danger of over-involvement is that the nurse may use the patient for her own emotional needs and her own feelings will dominate the relationship.

Some pointers to over-involvement on the part of the nurse include: preoccupation to the exclusion of other patients; resenting other nurses' relationships with the patient; taunting other staff with the assertion that she is the only one who understands the patient; ignoring the views of others on the nursing of the patient and making enquiries about the patient while off duty.

While accepting the dangers of over-involvement, it would be wrong for the nurse to remain detached and to try to convince herself that she has no feelings for the patients. Of course she does, she would not be human otherwise. It is better that she should accept involvement and attempt to discover what her feelings are, how they influence the relationship, and how she can come to terms with them for the maintenance of a satisfying and therapeutic contact. If there is no regular supportive staff group the nurse should seek the support of other team members.

Manipulation

Occasionally a patient may try to manipulate the nurse so that he may have his own way. The nurse should learn to recognise behaviour which is indicative of manipulation. For example, the manipulating patient may create situations to obtain her undivided attention. He may constantly flatter her. He will always agree with her, but may ridicule other staff, claiming that she is the only one who can understand and help him.

Constraints in relationship development

Sometimes it is difficult for the learner to develop a relationship with patients because of the nature of her training. The patient may be aware that the nurse will only be on his ward for a few weeks and this may hinder his involvement. The nurse must also learn to accept that she cannot have a close relationship with all the ward patients. She is not superhuman and such a relationship is not possible in a short period of time. Also, the nurse should not feel a failure if some patients do not accept her or make contact, this does happen and it is no fault of the nurse. If she has tried her best and discovered that she is getting nowhere with a particular patient, she should not take it personally. His refusal to accept her may be due to many factors. For example, he may have delusions of persecution against all nursing staff, or he may lack insight and not see the need for treatment and nursing care.

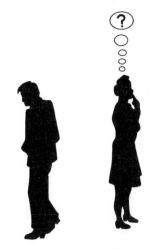

The nurse should not feel a failure if some patients fail to accept her. This does happen and it is usually no fault of the nurse

Fig. 6.2 Rejection

Friendship

Many psychiatric patients are friendless. Their illness may have prevented friendship or their long stay in hospital may have severed all links with old friends. Such patients may regard the nurse as a friend. However, this can only be a one-sided friendship since it would not be appropriate for the nurse to burden the patient with her personal problems. The patient will regard the nurse's friendship as a personal one and many demands may be made. The nurse should not resent these but learn to balance them in her overall relationship with the patients. It is usually helpful for the nurse to reduce the patient's demands by encouraging him to develop friendships with other patients, voluntary workers, League of Friends, visitors, pen friends and so on.

Dependence

Sometimes patients may become too dependent on a nurse. They may learn to expect her to make all their decisions for them when they may be capable of doing so for themselves. The nurse should be aware of this and slowly reduce the patient's dependence on her. She should learn to recognise over-dependence and gradually reduce the role of her relationship in the patient's life. She should encourage him to stand on his own and broaden the relationship to include more and more independent decisions and involve a wider range of personnel.

Staff relationships

The therapeutic effectiveness of the nurse's relationship with the patient does not exist in isolation from the other members of the staff caring team. It is essential for the recovery plan that all staff maintain harmonious relationships in the wider interests of the therapeutic environment and the patient's ultimate recovery.

It is pointless for the nurse to try and convince herself that she has a truly therapeutic relationship with the patient if, at the same time, she has an unco-operative attitude with, e.g., the ward doctor or occupational therapist. Equally, it is difficult for the nurse to maintain a therapeutic relationship if the ward sister or doctor constantly interferes with the nurse/patient relationship and undermines her efforts.

One-to-one relationships

With the recent increase in nurse therapy, nurses are called upon to form more specific relationships with individual patients. These relationships are similar to those used in psychotherapy and they involve a closer human contact. The nurse usually meets the patient at an appointed time and from these meetings an understanding develops between nurse and patient.

Transference

In transference relationships the patient projects his feelings and thoughts on to the nurse. He substitutes the nurse for some other person in his life and she may become the target for anger, hate, love, criticism or admiration.

Counter-transference

This is transference in reverse. With counter-transference it is the nurse who may project her feelings and thoughts on to the patient.

Relationship development

Points to consider
- Keep relationships professional rather than social
- Avoid being too personal
- Learn to recognise emotional involvement
- Do not take rejection too personally
- Accept the patient as an individual
- Learn to trust the patient
- Do not encourage over-dependence
- Do not try too hard to impress the patient
- Never ignore the patient
- Do not talk down to the patient
- Respect confidences and keep promises
- Always keep prearranged appointments

Note on relationships

A new development in psychiatric nursing is the use of different relationship techniques or strategies to deal with various patient problems. Such strategies can be operative on a one to one basis or imparted through behaviour therapy, milieu therapy or groups. Therapy groups in particular can be used to help patients with personality traits which cause interpersonal problems. As Gahagan (1975) pointed out, the growth of personal relationship groups is an important step forward in psychology.

Group work

This can be used to explore relationship strategies which nurses may deploy in dealing with the following patient problems:
1 Aggressive behaviour
2 Attention seeking
3 Unco-operative behaviour
4 Withdrawal
5 Obsessional handwashing

7
General Nursing Care

1 Activities for daily living

An important part of the nurse's duty is to help the patient to meet his needs. In normal health an individual performs a number of activities which are part of his daily life. These activities are necessary for a person's physical, psychological, social and economic functioning, and include feeding, breathing, elimination, personal cleansing, grooming, walking, talking, seeing, hearing, socialising, working, playing, relaxing and sleeping.

In normal health these activities are not a problem because the patient can perform them unaided. However, mental disorder may impede or distort the performance of essential activities and disrupt the patient's ability to function as an individual. Consequently, these activities become problems for the patient and the process of nursing must help him to resolve them.

2 Assessing activities

Each person is different and so his problems will be unique to him. Consequently, when planning care and treatment, the nurse must identify and assess the patient's needs as follows:

(a) Those he can perform unaided
(b) Those he can perform with limited help
(c) Those he cannot perform

The first two activities are concerned with self-help and may be seen as the patient's input to recovery. It is important for the patient's independence and self-esteem to encourage and permit self-help in so far as symptoms, treatment and nursing resources will permit. The patient will be dependent on the nurse for those activities which he cannot perform himself. The nurse should be aware, however, that the level of achievement in activities is not always static. For example, that for which the patient is dependent on others today, he may be able to perform by himself tomorrow.

3 Nursing care guidelines

Psychiatric patients may neglect their body needs and deteriorate physically. The following factors should receive attention:

Personal hygiene

Care of the body is commonly neglected. Evidence of neglect can be seen in the patient's failure to wash, bath, clean his teeth and attend to hair or nails. He appears to lack the interest, energy and ability to deal with everyday hygienic practices. It is necessary for the nurse to supervise personal hygiene and stimulate the patient to adopt good health habits. As the patient improves the nurse should encourage him to be responsible for his own hygiene.

Bathing. The patient should be encouraged to shower or bath as often as is necessary for cleanliness and general ease. The nurse must promote dignity and comfort by ensuring that the room is warm and private. Some patients need help and supervision. For example, new admissions, epileptic and suicidal patients, elderly and confused patients, and those who may fail to wash properly, such as schizophrenic, manic, deteriorated and obsessional patients.

Hairwashing. The hair should be washed with a suitable shampoo weekly. The nurse should encourage the patient to make use of the hospital hairdressing department for washing, cutting and styling.

Teeth. Each patient should have his own individual toothbrush and toothpaste or denture cleanser. The nurse must encourage the patient to brush his teeth on getting up in the morning, following meals, and before going to bed at night.

Nails. The nurse may have to attend to the patient's nail care but preferably the aim should be to encourage the patient to manicure his own nails.

Shaving. Male patients need to be encouraged to shave daily using either a safety blade razor or an electric shaver. It is the practice on many psychiatric wards for all blades to be accounted for as they are used.

Cosmetics and grooming. Many patients may look shabby; hair may be untidy and clothing stained. This makes it difficult to further rehabilitation because the patient may not be interested in how he appears to others. The nurse can do much to remotivate patients by boosting their ego through encouragement to wear make-up, have their hair styled, use deodorants, and brush their clothing.

Clothing. Patients should be encouraged to wear their own clothes in preference to institutional garb. Patients who cannot afford clothing should be referred to the social worker to seek a clothing allowance. Personal choice of clothing enables the patients to select styles and colours they like, and it encourages them to be more responsible for looking after them.

Patients who are unable to select clothing should be guided by the nurse to dress appropriately for the occasion and the season. Some patients require supervision to care for clothing and each individual should have his own locker. Plenty of time is allowed for good grooming and most hospitals provide dry cleaning, ironing, washing and mending facilities.

Food

In mental illness a variety of diet problems may occur: some patients may refuse to eat; some eat too much and some may 'cram' food or have table manners which are objectionable.

The onus is on the nurse to ensure that the patient receives an appetising and well balanced diet. Patients should be aware of the meal times, and their interest should be aroused by talking about food and menus. Patients' likes and dislikes are important factors and, where possible, 'food fancies' should be allowed for by a wide choice. Patients must be given plenty of time to prepare for their meals, especially to wash their hands and tidy up. The meal itself should be a pleasurable occasion. Each course should be served attractively and separately. The whole procedure should be unhurried, undisturbed and free from anxiety and disappointment. Those with special feeding problems may require individual nursing supervision (see Chapter 15).

Elimination. Individual bowel and bladder habits should be assessed. A daily record will help the nurse to build a picture of the patient's pattern. Common causes of constipation in psychiatric patients are drugs, diet, depression, senility and invalidism. To avoid or alleviate the condition it is important that patients are encouraged to include plenty of roughage and fluid in their diet and to take as much exercise as possible. The skin of incontinent patients should be washed with soap and water to prevent breaks. Retraining may be necessary. Patients preoccupied with bowel function who frequently request aperients should be reviewed by the doctor.

Exercise and posture. Many psychiatric patients exercise little and adopt incorrect posture habits; this applies particularly to depressed and long-term patients. The care plan should introduce the patient to work and leisure activities which will promote mobility, relaxation and posture. Resources for remedial therapy and physiotherapy should be utilised.

Physically ill patients

Psychiatric patients with physical illness may find it irritating to be restricted in this way, so the nurse must do everything necessary for physical recovery. She must reassure the patient and support him in coming to terms with his situation. She should keep the patient comfortable and prevent complications which may result from being bedfast. In addition to providing for the patient's basic physical needs, nursing care concentrates on the prevention of pressure sores, venous thrombosis, foot drop and chest infections. The nursing plan should also provide for special problems which may occur, such as pain, incontinence or paralysis.

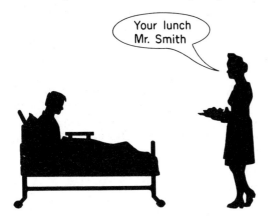

Fig. 7.1 Caring skills

Other needs

Social, psychological and economic needs are related to other chapters throughout the book. A summary of these includes: the need for acceptance and understanding; the need to feel secure;

the need for recognition and attention; the need for self-esteem; the need for love and friendship; the need for dependence/independence; the need to be occupied and the need for communication.

Special needs of dying patients

In addition to basic needs, e.g. diet, fluid, comfort, elimination, there are additional nursing problems associated with the physical and psychological process of dying. These include:

1 Physical changes

Loss of energy. The patient weakens and tires very easily. Drives are reduced and he is less able to help himself with basic functions such as washing, feeding and eliminating.

Motor system failure. When the power of movement fades the nurse should maintain correct limb positions, turn the patient frequently and avoid pressure from bedclothes.

Circulation. Peripheral circulation begins to fail, causing the skin to feel cold while internal temperature remains high. The patient may sweat and become restless. He should be kept cool and comfortable with light bedclothes.

Hearing and sight. These begin to fail. The patient can only see and hear what is near. The nurse and relatives should go close to the patient when attending to him.

Communication. This may be difficult but the nurse should ask the patient to raise his eyebrows or blink his eyes if he understands.

Awareness. As this may remain until the very end, the nurse must continue to give total care.

Pain. Fear of pain can be a persistent need in the dying patient. If injections are prescribed they may be ineffective when peripheral circulation fails, unless given intravenously.

Religious needs. As these are strong during the dying process, chaplains should visit frequently and the nurse should read from the Bible or prayer book if the patient requests.

2 Psychological changes

Emotional needs may vary but recognised stages to death include:

Initial shock. This may be accompanied by general shock sweating and fainting.

Denial and disbelief. The patient may react by denial, saying, e.g., 'It's a mistake'.

Anger. As the patient gradually realises the truth he may become angry, saying, for example, 'Why me?'. During this period he may resent people who are well and can be critical of everything the nurse does.

Bargaining. Some dying patients may bargain with God. For example, they may plead 'If you let me live another two years I promise this'.

Depression. The patient becomes quiet and may cry silently and refuse visitors. He needs time to meditate and become reconciled to giving up his loved ones. The nurse must allow him this.

Acceptance. This is the final stage and the patient is now more content and resigned to his situation.

The nursing plan must aim to help the patient through the different stages. The nurse should never leave the patient lonely or abandoned. She should always maintain his dignity and call his relatives to the bedside when death is approaching.

The question of whether 'to tell' or 'not to tell' the patient remains a dilemma. It will depend on the patient, and the doctor usually makes the decision.

Relatives will require help with their own emotions. When the patient dies it helps them to 'let it out' by crying. The nurse should comfort and hold them if necessary.

4 Nursing objectives

The psychiatric nurse should develop clear objectives when managing patient care. There may be a tendency on the part of some nurses to set objectives in general terms of helping the patient

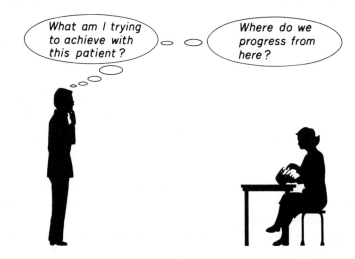

Fig. 7.2 Setting objectives

to get well and go home. This approach may be too vague however, because recovery is often a step-by-step affair with the patient's illness sometimes extending over several months or years.

The nursing care plan should include both short- and long-term objectives to help the patient and his nurses to know what they are working towards and to assess progress at any given time. Ward meetings should be used to co-ordinate the different objectives of the caring team to ensure continuity and prevent individuals working at opposites to each other.

5 Responsibility

Nursing care carries many responsibilities and loyalties which may be considered under two headings:

(a) The patients

It is the nurse's responsibility to administer treatments correctly, observe accurately, plan care programmes, record objectively, prevent accidents and so on. The nurse must execute the duties allocated to her by the senior staff and report back if she is unable to complete the tasks allocated. The nurse should be careful to avoid assuming responsibilities which are outside her scope or if she lacks competence to deal with them.

There are many occasions when the nurse will be required to make decisions and accept the consequences of her actions. She may be given individual responsibility for a particular patient, or a group of patients, which may involve her in emergency actions. For example, she may have to act in response to sudden unpredictable behaviour from a patient.

(b) The hospital

Employment in the hospital organisation bestows certain responsibilities on the nurse. She is an individual acting on the hospital's behalf in many matters such as injuries to the patient or to members of the public, maintaining confidentiality, collecting money and valuables for safekeeping, completing accident forms and eliminating fire hazards.

The nurse also has a responsibility towards the hospital in such matters as maintenance of hospital property, careful use of resources and conservation of energy. Lastly, the nurse has responsibilities towards other health members and towards her junior colleagues for their training and supervision needs.

6 Evaluating care

The nurse must constantly evaluate the effectiveness of the nursing care plan and of her own actions. Evaluation should relate to the success or failure of her objectives. For example, if evaluation shows that the patient's care plan failed to achieve objectives (such as the prevention of pressure sores or the forestalling of suicidal attempts), then the nurse should follow up and try to determine the reason for failure. On-going evaluation will help her to modify her care plan as progression or regression occurs.

Continuous feedback is necessary to provide information for others. It will help the doctor to evaluate the patient's response to treatment, therapy, leave of absence and so on.

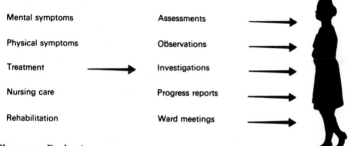

Fig. 7.3 Evaluation

Summary

It is helpful for nurses to use a scientific framework or model when delivering nursing care. The nurse should consider the patient as an individual, assess his problems, prepare a care plan to resolve these problems, implement the plan and evaluate progress. Nursing care is not a static activity; the patient will change from day to day and therefore the process must give continuity and remain open-ended. Nursing care must be relevant to each patient's problems and the nurse should think critically and objectively about the effects of her own actions and intervention (see Chapter 11).

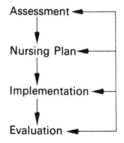

8

Basic Behavioural
Nursing Care

Patient behaviour

The psychiatric patient's behaviour is what he does. Sometimes this behaviour may be agreeable while at others it may be disagreeable. It includes his basic human actions, whether a peculiar way of eating, a habit of drying his hands on the bedcover, a persistent talking to voices no one else hears, or whatever.

In simplified terms we may say that there are two general types of behaviour: good or desirable behaviour and bad or undesirable behaviour. The former is agreeable to social functioning while the latter may be disagreeable in that it creates personal difficulties and barriers to social intercourse. For example, we could say that the patient who washes his hands and dries them with a towel would be behaving in a more desirable manner than a patient who continues to dry his hands on the bedcover, causing it to become wet and soiled.

Encouraging desirable behaviour

It is widely accepted that the nurse can do much to improve the patient's behaviour at a basic level. Her day-to-day involvement with the patient places her in a unique position to help him unlearn old patterns of behaviour and learn new ones. Each event which involves the nurse interacting with the patient is potentially capable of bringing about change in the patient's behaviour.

What is important for the nurse to realise, however, is whether the behaviour being encouraged is appropriate for the patient's recovery, for it has been demonstrated that nursing staff frequently reinforce a patient's bad or undesirable behaviour. For clarification, we will return to the above example of hand drying. If the nurse fails to correct the patient when he dries his hands on the bedcover, she may be silently condoning the undesirable act and worse still, her silent approval may be reinforcing the bad habit.

Behaviour and the long-stay patient

The long-term patient presents an intractable treatment problem in modern psychiatry. Many such patients are withdrawn, apathetic and show little initiative. They avoid social contact with other patients and many may not have spoken a word to anyone for several years. Their behaviour is odd and occasionally they may have aggressive outbursts or exhibit unco-operative attitudes by refusing meals, medication or other aspects of their normal routine.

Consequently, the nurse, through her relationship with the long-stay patient can be a positive element in his treatment and rehabilitation. Smart clothing, attractive wards, recreation, occupation and other therapeutic activities are also important but can mask the patient's continuing stagnation if a positive nursing approach is lacking.

The nurse's role provides her with the opportunity to interact with the patient almost every hour of his waking day. This means that the nurse is the prime mover in basic treatment through her close proximity to him. If the patient does not speak or lacks initiative, she is there to encourage him. It is this 'on the spot' position of the nurse which makes her the principal agent in making care and rehabilitation truly therapeutic.

Approval/disapproval

When improving behaviour, the nurse must learn to recognise the patient's efforts and to praise him when he responds. By doing so,

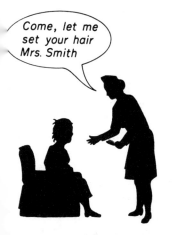

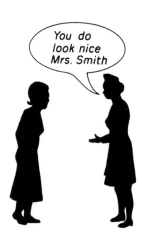

Fig. 8.1   Remotivating   Approval

the nurse is showing approval and thus giving further encouragement. It has long been recognised in psychiatric nursing how patients very often like to 'please' the nurse. This is a very positive factor in the nurse/patient relationship and can be used for effecting responses from the patient. Patients learn to adopt the correct habits in response to the nurse's approval as shown by her encouragement, praise, compliments and so on. When a patient makes the effort to brush his hair for the first time in many years, little comments such as 'You do look smart', 'very nice', or 'Well done', can go a long way towards encouraging the patient to repeat the behaviour.

It is equally important for the nurse to show disapproval towards undesirable behaviour from her patients. For example, when a patient is messy with his food or ignores his personal hygiene, the nurse must show some form of disapproval through an unfavourable expression or a comment such as 'That is wrong', or 'You must not make a mess'. Positive verbal reinforcement helps the patient to learn that his behaviour, though excusable on this occasion, is unacceptable for his eventual social functioning.

Specific behaviour modification

The techniques involved in behaviour modification are based mainly on the theories and experiments on learning carried out by notable names such as Pavlov, Thorndike and Skinner. Their experiments on animals showed how patterns of behaviour can be learned by repetition of certain stimuli. So far we have related some of these principles to show how the nurse can contribute towards shaping new learning through her hour-to-hour involvement with the patient's basic nursing care.

However, more specifically, the nurse may also be involved in behaviour treatment aimed to disrupt some of the unwanted and incapacitating habits found in many patients. In such cases, a more intensive technique is used to eradicate the undesirable habits or responses to specific objects or situations, in order to unlearn them, and to introduce new responses which are less incapacitating than those being extinguished.

Treatment programmes have been evolved to treat such conditions as obsessional states, phobic anxiety states, sexual problems and alcoholism. Many such programmes aim to modify certain behaviour by using positive and negative reinforcements to establish new responses. Similar techniques can also be used to treat chronic schizophrenics, patients with psychotic behaviour in general, children with behavioural disorders and the mentally handicapped.

Patients who require close day-to-day supervision such as for the toilet, meals and dressing, have shown considerable improvement as a result of nurses discouraging undesirable behaviour and encouraging other wanted behaviour.

Special programmes can be used which incorporate a reward system. The patient receives the reward when the target behaviour has been achieved and may then use it to obtain some privilege, e.g., buying cosmetics.

Nurses participating in treatment programmes must have a sound understanding of the psychological principles involved. If the programme is not carried out effectively it may not be therapeutic for the patient. Conversely, many nurses tend to achieve a high degree of job satisfaction and some may pursue a specialist course in therapy nursing (see Chapters 15 and 35).

Nursing care versus nursing behaviour

The nurse must learn to balance her roles as care agent and behaviour change agent. In some instances, with the newly admitted patient, the acutely disturbed patient, the severely depressed patient, the elderly sick person and the confused patient, e.g., the balance must be in favour of care; while in other instances such as the institutionalised patient, the neurotic patient, the recovering schizophrenic and the mentally handicapped patient, the balance will be in favour of behaviour change.

In the early stages of recovery the nurse is initially an observer, a doer, and a provider, when caring for the patient's physical needs. During this period her relationship with the patient is developed and out of this will grow her usefulness as a basic behaviour change agent.

The nurse's roles are complementary and the pace of shaping the desired behaviour should progress with each stage of recovery. At no time should it be enforced at the expense of the patient's physical well-being.

9
Introduction to Mental Disorder

Incidence

Approximately 5 per cent of the general population will require treatment for a mental disorder at some stage of their lives. Opinions vary but the conclusion from estimates is that as many as 20 per cent of patients attending general out-patient clinics and visiting general practitioners have an emotional basis to their complaint which calls for psychotherapy, social readjustment or other psychiatric help.

Forty per cent of the hospital beds in the National Health Service are occupied by mentally disordered persons. Though the number of hospitalised patients decreased by 64 000 from 1964 to 1982 (England and Wales), there remain approximately three per thousand of the general population receiving in-patient treatment for major mental disorder at any given time. This figure also includes geriatrics and the mentally handicapped. Over the same period the number of admissions (mostly readmissions) increased by 5000 and the total attendances at day hospitals doubled to over 2.5 million in 1981, and the total out-patient attendances were almost 1.75 million in the same year (*Facilities and Services of Mental Illness and Mental Handicap Hospitals*, DHSS, London, and Welsh Office, Cardiff, 1983).

Classification

Psychiatric classification is descriptive because the underlying causes of most mental disorders are unknown. In modern psychiatry opinions and approaches may differ but the following classifications are generally accepted in clinical practice:

1 The neuroses

These are conditions which are commonly caused by stress and result in extreme behaviour from the normal. They include *anxiety* and *phobic states, hysteria, reactive depression* and *obsessional-compulsive states.*

Insight and neuroses

'Insight' is the term applied to the recognition by a person that he is ill. Patients with neuroses may accept that they are sick but some will attribute this to a physical factor and totally ignore the real cause which may be psychological. People with neurotic illnesses are in touch with their environment and reality. They do not usually have gross personality deterioration or disintegration.

2 Functional psychoses

These are diseases which appear to have no physical disorder but usually show gross behaviour dysfunction. They include:

(1) *Mania* – an excitable, over-active state. The clinical types are hypomania and acute mania.

(2) *Manic-depression* – a despairing depression of the manic-depressive state which may also be known as endogenous depression.

(3) *Involutional Melancholia* – a specific agitated depression occurring in middle-aged persons.

(4) *Schizophrenia* – a serious illness which disturbs the thoughts and emotions. Abnormal behaviour, fantasising and withdrawal are features.

The clinical types of schizophrenia are:

(a) Simple schizophrenia – onset common in late teens and early twenties.

(b) Hebephrenia – common in young adults.

(c) Catatonia – excitement and stupor are features.

(d) Paranoid schizophrenia – more common in middle-aged patients.

(e) Chronic or long-term schizophrenia – applies where patients' schizophrenia has progressively crippled their personality and motivation. Many long-term schizophrenics are referred to as being institutionalised.

3 Central nervous system syndromes

These are psychotic conditions which are influenced by a physical disorder and are classified in relation to the cause of the underlying physical disorder. They may be acute or chronic and include:

(1) Degenerative conditions such as Huntington's chorea, Alzheimer's disease, Pick's disease, senile degenerative dementia, multiple sclerosis.

(2) Infections, e.g. acute toxic-confusion, meningitis, cerebral syphilis, encephalitis.

(3) Arteriopathic disorders, e.g. arteriosclerotic dementia.

(4) Brain tumours.
(5) Endocrine disorders, e.g. thyrotoxicosis, myxoedema.
(6) Chemical disorders, caused by drugs and alcohol.
(7) Anoxia.
(8) Trauma.
(9) Others, e.g. epilepsy, Parkinson's disease.

Insight and psychoses

Most psychotic persons are said to have no insight, i.e. the patient may insist that he is not ill, and that he has never felt better, when it is obvious to the observer that he is very disturbed.

Patients with psychotic diseases are unable to test and evaluate external reality and may show gross personality disintegration and behaviour dysfunction. They usually show a break with reality and do not always respond to their environment.

4 Other conditions

Some conditions do not fit readily into a neurotic or psychotic system of classification. Some may be classified as personality disorders or are simply referred to by their clinical name.

(1) *Mental handicap* – includes conditions such as Down's syndrome and cretinism. These states are present at birth or occur early in life (see Chapter 26).

(2) *Psychopathic or sociopathic states* – patients in this class are clinically recognised as aggressive, creative or inadequate.

(3) *Alcohol dependence* – persons addicted to alcohol may become mentally or physically ill from heavy consumption.

(4) *Drug dependence* – hard and soft drug addiction.

(5) *Anorexia nervosa* – dislike of food to the point of starvation.

(6) *Sexual disorders* – include conditions such as fetishism, voyeurism, transvestism, homosexuality, exhibitionism, impotence and frigidity (see Glossary).

(7) *Psychosomatic diseases* – physical disorders which are influenced by psychological factors, e.g. migraine, bronchial asthma and hypertension.

Causes of mental disorder

No specific single cause can be found for most mental conditions. In a minority of states (syphilis, e.g.) the cause is clearly due to a micro-organism but in other states, notably mania, schizophrenia and depression, a definite cause is not evident. In the absence of a known cause, theories abound to cover a whole range of suggestions relating to physical, chemical, environmental, psychological, inheritance and constitutional factors. Since a person's health is dependent on the social, physical and mental interaction, the cause of mental disorder may involve any or all of these factors.

1 Heredity

Genes are the elementary factor in heredity and there are hundreds of thousands in each of the 46 chromosomes (chains of genes) found in human tissue cells. Genes transmit the characteristics they control from one generation to another. Each gene has a basic chemical structure of deoxyribonucleic acid (DNA) which is seen as a functional region that maintains its identity, has a specific action, is capable of reproducing itself, and provides a code for the production of proteins (often enzymes) which speed chemical processes in cells.

A genetic heredity factor is described as dominant when a disorder can be transmitted by an abnormal gene carried by one parent only, e.g., in Huntington's chorea. A genetic heredity factor is described as recessive when a disorder can be transmitted only when both parents carry the abnormal gene.

Inheritance plays a part in some mental illnesses. For example, Huntington's chorea and some mental handicap conditions. In manic-depressive psychosis and schizophrenia, inheritance factors are thought to play a predisposing role.

2 Physical constitution

A person's body build has been linked to mental illness by the work of Kretschmer (1936). He divided body build into three main types:

   (a) *Pyknic build* – short neck, fat, with large trunk.
   (b) *Asthenic build* – skinny, lean, with little muscle or fat.
   (c) *Athletic build* – a muscular, athletic type of body.

According to Kretschmer, pyknic physiques were liable to manic-depressive illness and cyclothymic (mood-swings) traits, and the asthenic build was linked with schizophrenia, while epileptics were predominantly of athletic build.

Sheldon largely superseded Kretschmer's work by using photographic studies of three body types (endomorphs, ectomorphs and mesomorphs) which corresponded with Kretschmer's pyknic, asthenic and athletic types respectively. Sheldon linked body build with temperament rather than liability to develop mental illness.

3 Human development

Psychological, physical and environmental factors may be influential at any time during a person's development from infancy to old age. Important periods include the following:

Infancy and childhood. Faulty upbringing in the early years of life may lead to personality problems in later life. Bowlby (1951) showed that maternal deprivation in the first two years of life may lead to serious personality disturbance. Though Bowlby has since modified his views, parental attention and attitudes are still considered to be very important in helping children learn how to give and receive affection, deal with aggressive feelings and sex in a healthy way, and to develop relationships with others.

Adolescence. This can be conflicting and stressful for many young persons. Physical and psychological changes need to be come to terms with and the young individual will be striving for independence and acceptance but may be insecure and uncertain about his future role in life. Factors such as unemployment, educational worries, relationships with the opposite sex and so on, may complicate matters. Many temptations face adolescents and for some, promiscuity or turning to alcohol or drugs may be possible reactions. Free-floating anxiety is not uncommon and mental illnesses such as hysteria, early schizophrenia and anxiety states often show for the first time during late adolescence.

Marriage and children. Marriage is a new situation which makes new demands on both partners. Attitudes may differ regarding having children, or one insecure partner may seek dependency and make crippling emotional demands on the other.

Although marital problems may exist in many marriages, it is interesting to note that mental illness occurs more frequently among divorced, widowed and single persons.

Middle age. This period in life brings physical and psychological stresses which may be a burden for some. For example, women have to come to terms with the menopause and both men and women are faced with reduced physical prowess and attractiveness to the opposite sex. There may also be anxieties about health, impending retirement, career and education of children, and so on. For some people the whole situation may look bleak and the future uncertain. Involutional depression is an illness which is associated with this time of life.

Old age. There are many social and psychological factors associated with old age which may lead to breakdown. Physical and mental capacities may decline and loneliness, boredom and physical disability are realities for many. Depression, hypochondriasis, anxiety, paranoid ideas and degenerative diseases may occur in this age group.

4 *Work*

Certain occupations may cause some disorders, e.g. peptic ulcers, more than others. Also, the nature of a person's employment may place him at risk in terms of temptation to alcohol. Persons with mental illness may attribute their problems to over-work and stress but in fact it is usually some feature in the person himself which has caused the breakdown.

Some workers may be given responsibility they cannot cope with and others may lose their self-esteem from being passed over for promotion. We also have to consider the many repetitive jobs in industry which cause boredom and frustration at the expense of the individual's well-being.

A person's illness may be unrelated to his work but it may have a profound effect on his efficiency in the work situation. For example, an anxious person may strive competitively but later become ineffective as his anxiety advances, while a depressed worker will lose interest in his job and his colleagues.

5 *Organic*

Physical disorder arising in the brain or another part of the body may cause dysfunction of mental activity. For example, infections such as syphilis may cause general paralysis of the insane, and alcohol or hypoglycaemia can produce an acute confusional state. Also, degenerative processes may destroy brain tissue for no known reason and cause diseases such as multiple sclerosis and pre-senile dementia.

6 *Trauma*

Mild injuries to the brain may produce acute mental dysfunction, while more serious injury may cause dementia. In punch drunkenness, e.g., small repeated injuries to brain tissue incurred during a boxer's career may produce psychiatric symptoms. In some cases a person's mental symptoms may not be due to the organic effects of an injury but rather to the person's personality reaction to an injury, e.g., neurotic reactions, compensation neurosis.

7 Endocrine disorders

Thyroid gland deficiency may result in cretinism, affecting children, and myxoedema, affecting adults, whereas over-secretion of thyroxine causes thyrotoxicosis.

8 Chemical agents

The intake of drugs or alcohol in large amounts over a period of time may damage the nervous system and cause psychiatric reactions. In many persons however, the alcohol or drug dependence may only be a symptom of some underlying personality problem or major mental illness.

Classification of mental disorder

The World Health Organisation (1967) classification of Mental Disorders is as follows:

Psychoses

Senile and pre-senile dementia; alcoholic psychosis; psychosis associated with intracranial infection; psychosis associated with other cerebral conditions; psychosis associated with other physical conditions; schizophrenia; affective psychosis; paranoid states; other psychosis and unspecified psychosis.

Neuroses, Personality Disorders and other Non-Psychotic Mental Disorders

Neuroses; personality disorders; sexual deviation; drug dependence; physical disorders of presumably psychogenic origin; special symptoms not elsewhere classified; transient situational disturbance; behaviour disorders of childhood; mental disorders not specified as psychotic associated with physical conditions.

Mental Retardation

Borderline mental retardation; mild mental retardation; moderate mental retardation; severe mental retardation; profound mental retardation and unspecified mental retardation.

In the British Isles the term 'mental handicap' is now preferred (see Chapter 26). See also the terms used under The Mental Health Act 1983.

(Reference: see p. 277, International Classification of Diseases).

10

Behaviour and Mental Disorder

Because behaviour patterns vary with each psychiatric disorder, it is helpful for the nurse to recognise the variety of signs and symptoms which patients may present.

General appearance

Personal care. This is commonly neglected in many psychiatric disorders, particularly the schizophrenic, depressive, manic and demented patient. The patient may look neglected, untidy and lack interest in appearance and hygiene.

Bizarre dress. Manic patients may occasionally wear excessive make-up and dress in a bizarre fashion.

Nudity. In acute excitement and confusional states, patients may repeatedly remove their clothing.

Ritualism. In obsessional states some patients are ritualistic when dressing or undressing. Excessive repetitive washing of the body may also occur.

Facial expression. This may be alert, anxious, hostile or apathetic.

Catatonia. This peculiar state of muscular rigidity is found in some schizophrenic patients. The patient may remain mute and posture may be abnormal. *Flexibilitas cerea* (waxy flexibility) is evident whereby the patient's limbs may remain for lengthy periods in positions in which they are placed.

Specific behaviour

Over-activity. This is commonly seen in manic patients. They are constantly 'on the go'. They appear to be in a great hurry and have little time for rest or routine.

Aggression. Many mentally disordered patients show aggression more easily because they do not have the same sophisticated mechanism for controlling aggressive urges as they had prior to their illness. They may silently direct their aggression inwardly on themselves, or periodically may unleash a verbal or physical onslaught upon a person or property.

Retardation. This involves a slowing down of thoughts and actions. This is shown by slowness in activity and speech which sometimes reminds one of a television action replay. Retardation is commonly seen in severe depression and commonly affects the whole body and bodily functions.

Stupor. This describes a state whereby the patient is completely motionless with little response to stimuli. It may be seen in catatonic schizophrenia and severe depression. This stupor is not to be confused with the semi-coma type stupor found in medical conditions.

Compulsions. Some patients have impulses or movements which they feel compelled to carry out even though they may desire to resist them. This may show itself in frequent washing of the hands, repeated checking that the door is locked and so on. Sometimes these actions may be called rituals and are commonly seen in obsessional-compulsive neurosis.

Withdrawal. Not uncommonly the schizophrenic patient withdraws and cuts himself off from interaction. He may become apathetic and indifferent to persons and objects in his environment.

Speech patterns

Sainsbury (1974) deals with two main elements when considering speech: the form or structure of speech and the content of speech as revealed in conversation:

1 *Form of speech*

Acceleration of speech is found in states of excitement and over-activity. If over-activity is marked there may be a flight of ideas whereby the person speaking may jump from one topic to the other.

Retardation (see p. 67).

Blocking. Patients with schizophrenia may suddenly stop speaking in the middle of a conversation and, following a pause, they continue on the same topic or on a completely unrelated topic. Blocking occurs due to obstruction of the stream of thought and may also be referred to as 'thought blocking'.

Incoherence is when little or no sense can be extracted from speech. This occurs due to an extreme disturbance in association of ideas whereby fringe ideas impinge upon the mainstream of thought. In schizophrenic patients normal speech may become bizarre due to disturbances of ideas so that one is often unable to follow the patient's conversation. The term 'thought disorder' is used to describe acceleration retardation, blocking, vagueness in thinking and so on.

2 *Content of speech*

Disorder of the content of thought, often revealed in the patient's conversation, can provide valuable insight into the patient's preoccupations in a number of psychiatric illnesses.

Ideas of reference. These occur commonly in suspicious patients. The patient is convinced that conversations or events relate specifically to him. For example, when the doctor comes into the ward and talks to the charge nurse he is sure the conversation is about him.

Delusions. A delusion maybe defined as a fixed false belief which is not in keeping with the patient's level of knowledge and cultural group and which cannot be altered by objective evidence or logical argument to the contrary. Delusions are found in many conditions and may be associated with perceptive disorders such as illusions and hallucinations. There are many different types of delusions and they may be pleasing or terrifying to the patient.

(a) *Persecution or suspicious delusions* are very common in psychotic conditions and are observed in the patient who wrongly believes that people are hostile and that he will be affected in some harmful way. For example, one middle-aged male patient believed that the local police station had a special computer which kept interfering with his thoughts. He also believed that all the traffic lights in England had secret cameras hidden in them which were linked up to the police station so that no matter where he travelled the police were able to watch him. As far as the patient was concerned this was real to such an extent that he would often present himself at the police station and accuse them of these 'foul deeds'. Occasionally there is the inherent danger that patients who feel persecuted may attack those whom they believe to be responsible.

(b) *Delusions of grandeur* are delusions where the patient falsely believes that he is a very important person in terms of either wealth, status, power or birthright. For example, he may believe he is a millionaire, a film star or royalty. Delusions of persecution and grandeur are frequently found together. For example, another patient believed that he descended from royalty and that he was the rightful heir to the throne of England. He also believed that the Prime Minister of the day was persecuting him because he was a threat to his rule. Thus, paranoid and grandiose delusions coexisted.

(c) There are many other delusions such as *delusions of sin*, *delusions of unworthiness*, *delusions of poverty* and *nihilistic delusions*. Nihilistic delusions are morbid false beliefs about body disorder. For example, the patient may believe that he has no heart, that his insides are rotted away or his limbs are missing.

Hallucinations. These are mental impressions of sensory vividness occuring without external stimulus. Hallucinations may involve all senses, namely hearing (auditory), sight (visual), touch (tactile), smell (olfactory), and taste (gustatory). The 'voices' or auditory hallucinations are the most common of those experienced by psychotic patients.

Hallucinations may show in several ways. The patient may state frankly that he hears voices; he may be seen in a listening attitude, he may talk aloud as if answering someone, or his lips may be seen to move. The patient may respond to his hallucinations by being a passive listener or he may reply to them. Sometimes more active responses may be made to hallucinatory commands by instant obedience. Hallucinatory insults may lead to attacks on bystanders or damage to property.

Hallucinations signify a break with reality and are usually indicative of psychotic states such as schizophrenia, mania, and organic conditions. Hallucinations may also occur due to the toxic effects of drugs or alcohol.

Illusions. These are similar impressions to hallucinations but differ in that they depend on a misinterpretation of an external stimulus (i.e. an external stimulus is present but the patient misinterprets this as something else). For example, the coat hanging behind the door in a dimly lit room becomes a person lurking and waiting to strike out. Illusions are common in acute confusional states.

Illusions can easily be made to occur, as is amply demonstrated in entertainment by illusionists. In the figure below for example, the lines in A and B are equal in length but appear unequal due to the arrangement of the end lines.

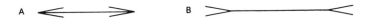

Fig. 10.1   Muller-Lyer Illusion

How the patient feels

The way the patient feels may have a marked effect on his behaviour, therefore the nurse should note his appearance in so far as it is indicative of his mood or emotional state.

Our feelings change in response to circumstances. In some situations we are happy but in others we feel sad or aggressive. It is normal under happy circumstances to feel and act happy, and here we can say that the affect or mood is appropriate. Abnormality can be assumed if our happiness is not consistent with, or is out of all proportion to, our circumstances.

Depression is a state of feeling which may vary from sadness or unhappiness to complete hopelessness and pessimism about the future.

Euphoria is a feeling of well-being, confidence and enthusiasm which is not justified by the surroundings.

Elation is a great feeling of well-being. The elated person is disproportionately cheerful, self-confident and optimistic, to a degree not justified by his surroundings.

Anxiety is a blend of fear, apprehension and uncertainty. Physical changes are associated with it, namely sweating, tenseness, tremors, palpitations, tachycardia, pallor, dryness of the mouth, lump in the throat and desire for elimination. Severe anxiety may be called panic.

Incongruous feelings are found in schizophrenia. For example, the patient may cry when it would be more appropriate for him to laugh or vice versa, thus the feeling is inappropriate or incongrous.

Apathy is commonly found in schizophrenia and is recognised as a lack of emotional response which is often severe and long lasting.

La belle indifférence may be seen in hysterical neurosis and shows itself as a bland lack of concern for distressing complaints or symptoms.

Confusion is used to describe a state of muddled thinking, lack of awareness of one's surroundings, and disorientation. The patient appears lost and mixed up. Questions may be answered irrelevantly and the memory and judgement impaired.

Sometimes elderly depressed patients with intellectual deterioration may appear confused when they are only inattentive and preoccupied.

Dementia is the term usually used to describe conditions with irreversible impairment of intellectual ability, memory and personality, due to diseases or damage to the brain.

In states of dementia there is a decline in intelligence, emotional changes and personality changes.

11

Nursing Process—A Problem Orientated Approach

Problem orientated care may be highlighted through the use of a systematic framework which recognises the patient as an individual and his need to be a participant in solving his own problems. Such a process should adapt to changes in the patient's condition and remain sensitive to his norms and expectations during care and treatment.

The framework for problem orientated care consist of four stages as follows:

(a) Obtaining information and conducting a critical assessment to identify problems which may be resolved by nursing care.

(b) Developing a written care plan, in consultation with team colleagues, which states the goals and actions for each problem.

(c) Implementing and monitoring the actions as prescribed in the care plan.

(d) Reviewing and reassessing problems to evaluate the effectiveness of care.

1   The assessment process

Psychiatric nursing history

A history should be established against a background of the patient's illness, personality, perception, family and social circumstances, with particular reference to the problems which precipitated hospitalization. A history is necessary in order to:

(1) Establish initial contact and rapport.

(2) Determine the type of person prior to breakdown.

(3) Establish the effect of mental crisis on the patient's physical, social, economic and psychological functioning.

(4) Identify specific problems and risk factors.

(5) Formulate priorities for nursing care.

(6) Identify the role of the patient and his family in the recovery process.

(7) Provide an information record which can be shared with other team members.

Data

This may be classified under the following headings:

(a) **Personal data**. Particulars regarding name, age, address, next of kin, reason for admission, family doctor, and so on.

(b) **Physical data**. Details about appearance, hygiene, grooming, diet, sleep, elimination, skin, mobility, posture, breathing, special senses, etc.

(c) **Socio-economic data**. Information regarding income, work skills, social skills, family, accommodation, etc.

(d) **Phychological data**. A picture of the patient's mental state in terms of personality, behaviour, perception, insight, communication skills, motivation, mood, attitude, interpersonal skills and so on. The nurse should assess the patient's general attitude to his mental health and mental problems.

(e) **Risk/Safety data**. Information to assess whether there are risks in terms of suicide, accidents, aggression, fits, drug side effects, dependency, pressure sores, infection, or other similar incidents.

(f) **Medical data**. Note the medical diagnosis, treatment investigations and community care as they may have implications for nursing care.

Interview technique

Initial contacts may influence the patient's willingness to co-operate in giving information. It is important to accept the patient, allow for individual differences and show understanding of behaviours. Examples of questions, illustrated later, should not imply that all such questions be put directly to the patient.

Guidelines for conducting an interview

1 Ensure privacy and reassure about confidentiality.
2 Assure the patient that the information being sought is necessary and important.
3 Exploring a certain line of enquiry should commence with open ended questions.
4 Show interest in the patient's answers.
5 Avoid technical jargon.
6 Avoid asking leading questions.
7 Pertinent information is obtained by direct forced choice questions.
8 Maintain eye contact.
9 Seek further clarification to ambiguous answers.

10 Allow the patient to complete statements without undue interruptions.
11 Respond to the patient's concerns whether they are immediately relevant or not.
12 Provide reinforcement with an occasional smile or expression.
13 Allow the interview to progress smoothly by avoiding delays in note taking or dialogue.
14 Do a summary at the end of the interview and allow the patient to discuss points and ask questions.
15 Arrange a date and time for a further interview if necessary.

Nursing diagnosis

Problems may be identified from a critical analysis of nursing observations and history data. It involves the nurse in making clinical judgements as to what she considers to be the relevant problems.

Mayers (1972) viewed problems as either actual, potential or possible. *Actual problems* are present at a point in time and can be identified (e.g. the patient is suicidal). *Potential problems* may be prevented by nursing actions (e.g. close observation to prevent suicidal attempts). *Possible problems* are not clearly identifiable and require further observation and study. Crow (1979) suggests that to assess the data the nurse should classify it into social, physical, emotional and economic categories.

Physical assessment

This should be a differential process as mental disorder may influence the activities for daily living and vice versa. The nurse should consider the following:

Emotions. Emotional states (e.g. anxiety) may cause headaches, diarrhoea, anorexia, sweating, palpitations and other complaints.

Behaviour. Psychiatric behaviour may distort the performance of physical activities such as exercise, washing, dressing and so on.

Physical Illness. Mental problems may prevent a physically sick person from seeking help. Assessment should not assume that all physical problems are a product of mental disorder.

Drugs and Alcohol. Physical problems may result from the side effects of drugs or alochol. For example, tremors, drowsiness, skin rashes, etc.

To highlight the assessment process further reference will be made to one physical activity as follows:

Nutrition. Assess eating habits. Likes and dislikes. Quality of diet. Weight. Domestic and social skills related to cookery and shopping. Cultural, religious or educational factors related to dietary habits. Psychiatric factors related to diet (e.g. anorexia, over eating, delusions, deteriorated habits). Physical factors related to diet (e.g. age, dexterity, false teeth, etc). Economic factors. Safety factors (e.g. epilepsy or confusion).

Social and economic assessment

The aim of social assessment is not to intrude unnecessarily into the patient's or family's life, but rather to be confidential and elicit the information needed to assess the social problems related to the person's illness, and ascertain the type of support he or his family require in the circumstances. A picture of the patient's family, dependants, accommodation, social contacts, occupation, income and general level of domestic, social and work skills and factors leading to admission should be established.

Psychiatric assessment

Eliciting the pertinent mental health problems may depend on the nurse/patient relationship and much will be learned from interactions and observations. Initial assessment should identify acute problems which require urgent attention.

It will be necessary to differentiate between behaviour which is part of the patient's illness as opposed to behaviour which is part of the person's personality and life style. The nurse should understand the limitations in attaching psychiatric labels to patients in a process which promotes individualised care.

To highlight the psychiatric assessment further, reference will be made to three mental factors as follows:

1 Personality. Establish the type of person the patient was prior to breakdown and note present traits such as whether he is quiet, solitary, outgoing, moody, anxious, obsessional, shows immaturity, or is suspicious, etc. Observe his general intelligence and his attitude to mental health, interests, hobbies and interactions. Assess self esteem and general level of coping resources.

2 Perception. Note perceptual functioning and describe errors such as delusions, hallucinations or illusions. Assess the effect of perceptual errors on behaviour. *(cont. on p. 79)*

Illustrated Nursing History and Assessment

Name: SARAH TOUGHY   **Age:** 31 years
Diagnosis: ANXIETY AND DEPRESSION

Classification	Comments
Physical	
Personal hygiene	Untidy appearance. Unkempt and neglects personal
Diet	hygiene
Elimination	Physically inactive but no mobility handicaps.
Skin	Has difficulty getting off to sleep.
Mobility	Poor appetite. One light meal and several cups of
Breathing	coffee per day.
Special senses	Poor perception of physical needs and health.
Aids	Underweight. Smokes 30 cigrettes per day.
Sleep	
Pain	
Socio-economic	
Family	Separated from husband over three years ago.
Work skills	Husband works overseas. No communication. Lives
Income source	with her mother in a private house in middle class
Accommodation	residential area. No accommodation problems.
Home environment	Three children at school aged 8, 6 and 5 years.
	Unemployed. Lives on social security. Not motivated to
	establish independence from her mother
Psychological	
Personality	Quiet and reserved. Low self esteem. Poor motivation
Behaviour	for self help. No wish to find employment. Mother does
Perception	most of the domestic management. Depressed, an-
Insight	xious mood. No personal friends. Poor social mixer.
Communications	Lacks confidence in social situations and fears failure in
Motivation	personal relationships. Longstanding, mental health
Mood	problems. One previous admission for depression 4
Attitudes	years ago. Intermittent treatment as an outpatient
Interactions	during the last 6 years.
Social skills	
Risks	
Suicide	Morbid thoughts and pre-occupation with depressive
Aggression	ideas. Feels she is a failure and a burden on her mother.
Accidents	Regard as medium suicide risk. Submissive, non-
Dependency	assertive attitudes. Feels inadequate. Regard as a
Constipation	medium dependency risk. Constipation may result from
	chemotherapy.
Medical	
Reason for admission	Reactive depression and anxiety with suicidal ideas.
Diagnosis	Anti-depressant therapy and psychotherapy. Routine
Treatment	physical examination and investigations. To be inter-
Investigations	viewed by social worker and community nurse.
Community care	Has been receiving supportive care from community
	psychiatric nurse over past 3 years.

Nurse's signature . . . .

Illustrated Care Plan—1
Name: SARAH TOUGHY

Date Defined	Nursing Goal	Nursing Actions and Activities Guidelines	Review Date
2.7.82	Establish rapport and enlist co-operation from the patient to develop a positive participative attitude to her problems	Develop a continuing one-to-one relationship. Give initial education and orientation about illness symptoms, treatment and care programme. Discuss nursing care plan and other treatment prescriptions with the patient and relative.	9:8:82
2.7.82	Reduce anxiety and preoccupation with illness.	Give crisis support and reassurance as required. Individual counselling, alternate days ×$\frac{1}{2}$ hour. Measure anxiety levels and monitor daily. Discuss positive feedback from investigations.	Review daily
2.7.82	Protect patient from initial stresses and promote a positive mental outlook and occupation.	Observe reactions and note risks. Involve in diversional activities morning and evening. Introduce to relaxation classes daily.	Review daily
2.7.82	Promote good health habits, in diet, exercise, breathing, sleeping.	Give advice on health education and smoking. Encourage daily exercises. Discuss sleep-coping resources and maintain sleep record. Give normal diet and food fluid extras. Record daily fluids and weigh weekly.	Review daily
2.7.82	Establish motivation for self-help in personal hygiene, grooming and domestic management.	Supervise daily washing and grooming. Reinforce positive responses. Appointments with beauticians twice weekly. Attend domestic therapy dept. twice weekly.	Review daily
2.7.82	Promote self esteem and confidence in relation to personal relationships, social situations and decision making.	Participate in group therapy and psychodrama. Innovate assertive therapy and reality confrontation exposure on a continuing basis. Develop coping resource learning. Develop social skills learning.	Weekly review meeting
14.7.82	Establish independence in relation to mother, work and accommodation.	Participate in work skills learning twice weekly. Introduce to occupational therapist, disablement resettlement officer and the community psychiatric nurse.	Weekly review meeting
14.7.82	Promote understanding of treatment perspectives.	Administer drugs and other treatments as per treatment prescription. Observe drug action and reaction.	Review daily
14.7.82	Progressive orientation towards discharge.	Evaluate progress towards discharge and assess follow-up requirements.	Weekly review meeting

Nurse's signature . . . . **Date** . . . .

Illustrated Care Plan—2

Name: JOHN SMITH
Age: 58 yrs **Date of Admission:** 1950
              Diagnosis: SCHIZOPHRENIA
                      Continuing Care Patient

Date	Problem	Action	Review Date	Progress
10.2.82	Disregards his personal hygiene.	Establish regular habits. Reinforce positive responses.	1.3.82	Shows interest in personal hygiene but this falls off if not supervised. Responds well to prompting.
10.2.82	Silent and uncommunicative.	Each nurse must encourage conversation. Greet patient each day. Never miss opportunities to speak and do not ignore. Reinforce responses.	1.3.82	Long periods of silence remain. John will reluctantly answer back when nurses insist on an answer. Request nurse therapist to assess this problem further.
10.2.82	Withdrawn and solitary.	Create interactive situations. Show, interest in John and participate with him in social and ward activities. Praise effort. Reinforce positive responses.	10.3.82	Will not enter into social or mixing situations of his own accord. Will participate when prompted by staff. Does respond to his sister during her weekly visits.
10.2.82	Devoid of interest for current news and events.	Daily reality orientation on day, date, month. Read daily paper headlines. Encourage John to watch the television news each day. Discuss news items, cost of living, etc.	10.3.82	Improvement noted in this area. John is now aware that he is living in the year 1982. Reads the daily paper headlines and appears to show an interest in the news. Expose more to group pressure.
10.2.82	Poor posture. Holds head and shoulders forward when sitting and walking.	Teach and encourage patient to adopt correct posture when sitting and walking.	10.3.82	Adopts correct posture when prompted by nursing staff. Further prompting and reinforcement necessary to maintain progress.

3 Motivation. Note general motivation regarding personal care, work, socialization and desire to get well. Observe whether re-education or remotivation is necessary. How much support will he require? What is his learning speed and how might he respond to incentives. Note ambitions and interests. Assess his general level of assertiveness and of independence.

2 Planning care

The Care Plan is the written prescription for the composite nursing actions which require implementation to solve or reduce the problems highlighted by the assessment process. When writing the care plan consideration should be given to nursing actions and planned activities most suited to the patient (see pp. 76—78).

Guidelines for completing a care plan

1. Commence with prescribing actions for actual problems.
2. List priorities.
3. Decide timing. How frequently must actions be performed and evaluated?
4. Relate timing to existing resources.
5. Relate prescriptions to existing resources and staff skills.
6. Prescribe preventive actions for potential problems.
7. State goal for each problem.
8. State review date for each problem.
9. Consider method of evaluation.
10. Discuss care plan with the patient and establish his role and contribution.
11. A team care plan may be used. Team prescriptions should be formulated at a team meeting and each member of the team should be aware of his role and contribution.

3 Evaluating nursing care

This is an on-going process to determine whether nursing prescriptions are being implemented and whether they are meeting the stated goals. Observations, team meetings and progress notes should build up a picture of the patient's response to nursing care, treatment and rehabilitation. New prescriptions or discontinuations should be highlighted. The patient's views should be included.

The effects of nursing care programmes, together with the impact of the care environment, must be evaluated and the necessary change or research implemented because they are implicit in the process of psychiatric nursing.

Feedback as an evaluation tool

Failure to develop constructive mechanisms to highlight feedback values may result in the repetition of low care standards. This may be due to misunderstanding of patient care in terms of effectiveness, expectations, problem behaviours, incidents and so on.

The outcome of some nursing actions can be measured using instruments (such as the clinical thermometer) while the outcome of other actions may rely on either the nurse or the patient's feelings, opinions, observations and interpretations.

Background Information

Initial evaluation should result from the monitoring of care programmes as follows:

1 Are all actions implemented according to the care plan?
2 Is focus being maintained on the patient's problems?
3 Are reviews and progress notes up-dated?
4 Have all problems been validated by the patient?
5 Are there deficiencies in resources which impede implementation?
6 Make a comparative analysis of the current state of the problem with the initial assessment.

Specific evaluation

Example 1

Initial assessment prescription	Evaluation feedback	Findings re-assessment	Review recommendations
Intense anxiety, inability to relax. Pulse 140. Blood Pressure 170/110. Muscles tense, restless. Introduce to relaxation classes and diversional therapy. Reassure and give explanations.	Study pulse and blood pressure charts. Observe progress notes. Note views at review meeting. Discuss with patient.	Pulse and blood pressure normal. No restlessness. Muscles relaxed. Still feels tense in exposed situations.	Reduce reassurance but support in threatening situations. Continue with diversional therapy and relaxation. Commence anxiety coping resource learning.

Example 2

Initial assessment prescription	Evaluation feedback	Findings re-assessment	Review recommendations
Expressing suicidal thoughts. Keep under continuous observation. One-to-one relationship.	Analyse progress notes. Staff review meeting. Discuss with patient.	No evidence of suicidal thoughts.	Reduce frequency of observations. Continue one-to-one relationship.

Worksheet for nurse learners—1

Patient's Name . . . .   Ward. . . . .

Date Commenced . . . .

Nursing Assessment. Highlight two current problems from an analysis of observations and data relating to any patient. Give explanations for your final judgements and conclusions.

Nursing Care Plan. Specify the nursing actions for these problems and state the expected outcome.

Implementation. Describe how you would maintain focus on the patient's problems when instituting care.

Evaluation. Identify methods of evaluation. How would you validate your evaluations? Re-assess the problem from an analysis of your evaluation.

Worksheet for nurse learners—2

Study the following psychiatric nursing interventions and identify problems which may be reduced or resolved by their use. The first one has been done for you:
Nurse—Patient relationships. This is a core intervention which has a key role to play both on a one-to-one and group basis for all psychiatric problems.

Reassurance. Counselling. Communication skills. Observation. Supervision. Health education. Safety. Habit training. Reinforcement. Self-help learning. Coping resource learning. Domestic skills learning. Social skills learning. Remedial therapy. Diversional therapy. Work skills learning. Economic skills learning. Reality therapy. Assertive training. Relaxation therapy. Group therapy. Psychodrama. Problem solving therapy. Crisis therapy. Restraint.

Research in psychiatric nursing

There are many patient problems which are intractable, despite the application of current psychiatric nursing interventions. Research must be carried out to increase our knowledge and understanding of their nature and with a view to developing other methods of effective care.

12

Anxiety Neurosis and Anorexia Nervosa

Note on neurosis

Neurotic individuals may be regarded by others as socially desirable and useful citizens. They tend to be moral, reliable, responsible, truthful and conformist. Their thought and behaviour tend to be inhibited and though they want to love and to feel loved, they are emotionally insecure and sensitive to the criticisms of others. They may be ambitious people but feel inferior, inadequate and dissatisfied with themselves. They are frequently anxious, tense and worried, and may have grave doubts and fears for the future. Since their suffering is largely internal they do not usually appear grossly abnormal to others but inwardly they may experience a wide range of physical disturbances.

Neurotic patients are usually inhibited, sensitive and lacking in confidence. There may be outward signs of anxiety, tension, or fearfulness, such as a tremor of the hands or voice or a marked startled reaction to unexpected sounds. Many also experience agitation and insomnia.

Many people are affected by neuroses and form a large proportion of people presenting themselves to general practitioners. The physical symptoms of which they complain may cause the illness to be mistaken for a physical one. Though neurotic patients will accept medical help they are sometimes reluctant to accept that their illness has an emotional basis. On the whole they are more likely to be treated at home or in out-patient clinics, but, for some, admission to hospital is necessary.

Anxiety states

Normal anxiety

Most people feel anxious before important events or when faced with grave risks. A man may be terrified by sudden danger. He may experience anxiety prior to stressful occasions such as examinations, interviews and public speaking. This is a natural reaction and disappears when the anxiety-provoking event is over. In an anxiety state, however, there is an irrational feeling of anxiety which is prolonged beyond the time of emergency or in the absence of any justifiable cause.

Acute anxiety

Onset

Acute anxiety is usually precipitated by some stressful event such as an unexpected bereavement, marriage crisis, serious accident or disaster.

Clinical picture

The patient experiences fear and apprehension. There is an excessive secretion of adrenaline which produces dilation of the pupils, profuse sweating, tachycardia, rise in blood pressure, pallor, fainting, dry mouth, giddiness, gooseflesh and rapid breathing. Diarrhoea, frequency of micturition, nausea, tremors and loss of appetite may occur. When the acuteness passes the patient may remain in a sub-acute state with symptoms of headaches, fatigue, insomnia, and inability to relax.

Chronic anxiety

Some patients may complain of constant feelings of anxiety, the severity of which may wax and wane without ever completely clearing up. They are chronic worriers many of whose worries centre round their physical and mental health. For example, the patient may believe that the physical changes in his body (produced by worry) are really due to some disease or other. His fatigue, loss of appetite and weight, insomnia, palpitations and headaches, support this belief. The patient has difficulty in accepting that his symptoms are psychological and not physical.

The patient may fear that he has heart disease, cancer, or that he is dying or going insane. The patient is usually tense, strung-up and unable to relax. His sleep may be disturbed by nightmares and he may wake up with a start to find he is shouting and drenched in sweat.

Irritability, depression, and inability to concentrate are usually marked, memory and judgement suffer and some patients feel exhausted and lose their sense of enjoyment and interest.

Phobic anxiety

Some patients may be anxious about some specific object or situation. Specific fears of this nature are called 'phobias'. For example, patients who are claustrophobic are afraid of being shut up in a closed space, and may be unable to go into a train or a cinema; in a room they may have to have the door kept open. When confronted by their phobia they panic and show acute anxiety.

There are many phobias and they may be classified as those relating to fears associated with insects, snakes and dirt, or diseases such as cancer, and those which are situational, such as fear of heights (acrophobia), fear of open spaces (agoraphobia), fear of closed spaces (claustrophobia).

The patient knows that these objects or situations are not really dangerous but he is unable to do anything about the irrationality of his fear. He may feel compelled to avoid situations or objects in an attempt to evade the acute anxiety and fear which exposure would cause.

Differential diagnosis

Anxiety neurosis must be differentiated from other mental conditions and physical illness. The features of other illnesses may resemble an anxiety state, e.g., thyrotoxicosis, peptic ulcer, heart disease, schizophrenia and involutional melancholia. Also, anxiety may be a symptom of other diseases (both physical and psychiatric) such as depression, hysteria, schizophrenia, organic brain syndromes, confused states, alcoholism, drug dependence and psychosomatic disorders.

Management and treatment

Out-patients

Most patients with anxiety neuroses are treated as out-patients and do not require hospitalisation.

(1) The patient's general practitioner may provide symptomatic treatment by prescribing minor tranquillisers such as: (i) chlordiazepoxide (Librium); (ii) diazepam (Valium); (iii) night sedative if necessary e.g. nitrazepam (Mogadon).

(2) A social worker and/or health visitor may be deployed to help with social or family problems if this is thought necessary.

(3) Serious cases may be referred to a specialist at an out-patient

clinic. Treatment may continue from the out-patient clinic or the patient may be given more support by attendance at a day hospital.

In hospital

Serious cases may require a period in hospital removed from the turmoil of everyday life. This gives the patient an opportunity to take stock of his illness and direct his resources to recovery. The treatment plan may include:

(1) Rest. Initially the patient may be fairly exhausted from the lack of proper sleep. For the first few days the patient may rest in bed and be given a hypnotic at night such as nitrazepam (Mogadon), 5 – 10 mg.

(2) Considering the optimum environment, a psychiatric unit or short term ward is most suited for this patient.

(3) Drugs. (i) Chlorpromazine (Largactil), up to 300 mg daily may be necessary for patients who are acutely preoccupied with symptoms. (ii) Diazepam or chlordiazepoxide to promote relaxation.

(4) Behaviour therapy. Desensitisation for specific anxiety (see Chapter 15).

(5) Psychotherapy. This helps the patient to understand his illness. He is helped to examine his symptoms and is encouraged by the therapist. Listening, reassuring, explaining and suggesting are important (see Chapter 35).

(6) Occupational and recreational therapy. These take the patient's mind off his problems and help him to feel a little better. They give satisfaction and prevent the patient from getting bored and preoccupied with his illness. They involve him with other patients and members of the caring team. They provide exercise and promote appetite and sleep.

(7) Relaxation therapy. Used with or without drugs to help very tense patients.

Nursing care

The nurse should:

1 Promote the patient's physical needs in terms of diet, rest, exercise and fresh air and give attention to hygiene and appearance.

2 Reassure. The nurse will be the primary agent in reassuring the patient. If physical symptoms are present, she should explain, in simple terms the physiological effects of anxiety. She should not tell the patient to pull himself together.

3 Observe. Watch and report progress and effects of treatments.

Note the patient's complaints and remember that these may not always be psychological – anxious patients can have something really physically wrong, just as any patient can.

4 Attempt to divert the patient's mind from his worries by changing the topic of conversation or encourage him to follow an interest or activity.

5 Encourage relaxation and contact with other staff and patients (e.g. group activities, music appreciation, games and other exercises).

6 If a panic attack occurs, give the patient her full attention and promote his confidence in her by dealing competently with the situation. She should avoid uncertainty in her own actions.

7 Maintain a calm, stress-free ward and prevent the patient's anxiety from affecting the atmosphere. Stay close to the patient during the crisis periods.

8 Out-patient and community psychiatric nursing support following discharge.

Anorexia nervosa

People with anorexia nervosa are underweight and emaciated through persistent refusal of food. Characteristically they behave as if they have lost their appetite. However, this is more a case of wilful starvation as the loss of appetite, in the sense of never being hungry, is not a central feature. Instead, an anorexic may at times be very hungry. In reference to this condition, Crisp (1976) coined the term 'weight phobia' to describe an attitude found in anorexia nervosa whereby the sufferer sees normal eating as leading to a gain in weight. Anorexia nervosa therefore is essentially about weight. The anorexic may suffer due to starvation and thinness, but compared with putting on weight it is seen as a lesser evil.

The majority of sufferers are adolescent girls and young women. About 1 in 20 are males.

Clinical features

1 Abnormally low body weight; at least 10 % below norm.
2 Amenorrhoea for *three* consecutive months.
3 Active refusal to eat.
4 Growth of fine downy body hair (lanugo) may be apparent.
5 Low blood pressure and basal metabolic rate.
6 Cold and cyanosed extremities.
7 Emaciation and anaemia.

8 Distorted body image.
9 Irritability, restlessness, insomnia and hostility.
10 Depression and obsessional traits may be present.

Diagnosis

1 History of behaviour which ensures a loss of weight. That is, avoiding food, self-induced vomiting, and excessive exercising. Occasional bouts of over-eating may feature.
2 Morbid fear of becoming fat and a determination to remain abnormally thin.
3 An implacable attitude that overrides hunger, admonitions and threats.
4 No evidence of mental or physical illness which accounts for the anorexia and weight loss.
5 Evidence of amenorrhoea, lanugo, uncontrolled gorging of food and vomiting.

Causes

Variations and explanations as to the nature of anorexia nervosa are considerable. A general view of causes include:
1 Personal conflict and emotional turmoil resulting from the hormonal and psychological changes in puberty and adolescence.
2 Vigorous dieting and slimming for cosmetic reasons.
3 Interpersonal stresses and anxiety about figure and sexual development.
4 Dysfunction in family relationships.

Aim of treatment

1 Restore normal weight and adequate balanced diet.
2 Support and readjustment to diminish food, figure and weight preoccupations.
3 Help the patient to develop worthwhile goals and mobilise alternative ways of coping with emotional conflicts and personal relationships.

Treatment plan

A combined physical and psychological approach is necessary.

Physical

1 Rest in hospital under specialist supervision.
2 Chlorpromazine (largactil) 150 mg three times daily. This has a stimulating effect on appetite.

3 Diet—a firm persistence on eating a well balanced diet.

Psychological

1 Psychotherapy and group therapy.
2 Behaviour therapy. A planned programme is devised in which rewards (reinforcement) are made contingent on either weight gain or satisfactory eating. Weight or food targets are explained fully to the patient (see Chapter 15).

Follow-up Treatment. Relapse following discharge is common. Treatment may continue following discharge from hospital. For example, behaviour programmes may be continued with the support of the family. Family therapy may be necessary to restructure the family relationships.

Nursing care

A nursing plan should be designed following an assessment of the patient and medical treatment regime. The following nursing interventions are usually necessary:
1 *Nurse—patient relationship strategies* such as support, counselling, reassurance, prompting, reality confrontation and supervision of food intake.

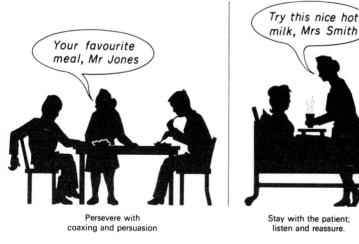

Your favourite meal, Mr Jones

Try this nice hot milk, Mrs Smith

Persevere with coaxing and persuasion

Stay with the patient; listen and reassure.

Fig. 12.1 Anorexia   Insomnia

2 Observation and recording of food intake, weight, temperature, pulse, respiration and elimination.
3 Rest and conservation of energy to prevent further weight loss.
4 Encouragement to meet weight or food targets.
5 Social and *expressive therapy* to reduce anxiety, irritability and boredom.

Evaluation of care

The caring team should *monitor* treatment and nursing care. Record charts should be analysed; weight records in particular will offer a guide to care effectiveness. Regular review meetings should take place for discussion on feedback and evaluative purposes. The patient's and relatives' views and attitudes should be considered.

(See References: Crisp (1976) and Dally (1979), p. 287).

13
Obsessional-compulsive Neurosis

Normal obsessions and compulsions

Many children step between the cracks on the pavement or touch the railings of a fence on their way to school. Many adolescents and adults may allow the words of a catchy tune to be repeated in their thoughts. Also, many adults may show some repetitive behaviour such as double checking if the gas taps are turned off, that the back door is locked, and so on. Again, many people at work will show obsessional traits: the nurse will check that she has administered the proper drug, the clerk that he has added up his figures correctly and so on. None of these people is inconvenienced by these little traits and they cannot be regarded as being abnormal.

Obsessional-compulsive neurosis

In this condition the patient is compelled to think or behave repetitively and cannot prevent himself from doing so. He may regard his thoughts and actions as unreasonable and ridiculous, but they produce such anxiety and guilt that he cannot dismiss them or give them up; his anxiety and agitation increase if he tries to stop thinking or doing what he feels he has to.

Symptoms

Obsessional thoughts. These may be of an unpleasant nature: blasphemous, aggressive or sexual, which continually run through the mind. Some patients may be obsessed with thoughts of being in some way dirty while others may be obsessed with numbers and feel compelled to write them down. Persons obsessed with thoughts of death may tick off every minute of the day.

Obsessional impulses, or compulsive acts. These may take a variety of forms. For example, an obsessional fear of germs or dirt may lead the patient to perform washing rituals.

One middle-aged woman was obsessed with the idea that she might become contaminated with cancer and spread this to her

husband. Consequently, she felt compelled to bathe her body nine
times each day using a fresh box of tissues on each occasion. She
changed her underclothes nine times a day and if interrupted, she
had to start all over again. What was even more pathetic about this
case was that she involved her husband in some of these rituals. As a
loved one he did not like refusing her requests and, in consequence,
she was making her husband's life miserable as well as her own.
Though this lady realised that what she was doing was absurd and
expensive, she was unable to prevent her actions.

Resistance to such compulsions results in increasing tension and
eventually the acts are carried out. Many patients become agitated
and depressed by their symptoms, and this in turn worsens their
condition.

Causes

Among the causes of obsessional neurosis the following are
important:
(a) Heredity. About one third of the parents and one fifth of the
siblings of obsessional patients have prominant obsessional traits. It
is likely that the patient would have been exposed to undue strict-
ness, regular habits and high moral standards during childhood.
(b) Physical factors. Obsessional neurosis may occur for the first
time following a head injury, infection or other organic brain
disease.
(c) Psychological factors. Conflicts and stresses between our moral
standards and the more primitive sexual or aggressive urges are
thought the basis for some obsessional neuroses.

Obsessional personality

Some obsessional neurotic patients may have had a previous
personality which was very rigid. They are the type of person you
may 'set your watch by'. They do things at a fixed time each day,
are excessively neat, meticulous in their work, check and recheck
detail and live by routine. It is important to note, however, that
many persons with this type of personality never have a
breakdown, while many obsessional patients may have no history
of such a personality.

Differential diagnosis

Obsessional symptoms may occur in many different kinds of
mental illness and many normal obsessions may become more
prominent during times of stress or ill-health. Neither of these

cases amounts to an obsessional neurosis. Also, some obsessional neurotic patients' behaviour and ritualism may be so bizarre and far-fetched that they may be wrongly diagnosed as schizophrenic. Obsessional acts may mask some diseases such as schizophrenia, depression and anxiety states.

Management and treatment

The treatment of obsessional neurosis will vary in method and result. Sometimes spontaneous remissions may occur, but on balance, obsessional states are notoriously resistant to treatment. Milder cases may be treated on an out-patient basis. The more incapacitating cases require admission to hospital. Treatment may include:

(1) Psychotherapy. This may give disappointing results, but where the symptoms are thought to relate to emotional conflict, frequently gain may come from this approach.

(2) Psychoanalysis. This fares no better than psychotherapy but it may be given a chance to get results (see Chapter 35).

(3) Drugs. Sedatives may help some patients to face situations which give them specific troublesome symptoms: (i) diazepam or chlordiazepoxide may be given to relieve the tension which is a common problem for the patient; (ii) antidepressant drugs such as imipramine may be given if depression is present.

(4) Electroconvulsive therapy (ECT). This may be used for the depression associated with the neurosis (see Chapter 34).

(5) Occupational therapy. This is very useful for occupying the patient and reducing the opportunity for him to practise his acts.

(6) Recreational therapy. Through this the patient is helped to relate, relax and enjoy himself.

(7) Behaviour therapy and deconditioning techniques. These sometimes give encouraging results in more specific phobic states. They are aimed entirely at symptoms with the aim being to eliminate them so that the patient can lead a fairly symptom-free life.

(8) Pre-frontal leucotomy. This may be used as a last resort in long-standing cases where there is severe agitation.

Promoting understanding

The patient's obsessional symptoms tend to be more tolerable in a calm, well-ordered ward environment. The nurse should attempt to reduce the patient's anxieties and fears using the techniques described on p. 16. It is important to avoid making too many demands on the patient. Discussion, explanation, and understanding of his problems will help him to become more relaxed. In mild cases the patient can be helped to understand that his compulsions are not harmful and if he can learn to be less anxious about them, he will be able to live a comparatively normal life. The nurse must also protect the patient from humiliation as other patients may ridicule his 'annoying' rituals.

Relieving symptoms

In severe cases the patient's acts are very incapacitating. The choice facing the nursing team is often a simple one of either:
  (a) Allowing the patient freedom and time to perform his ritual, or
  (b) Implementing a workable timetable aimed at reducing the time and opportunity for carrying out the obsessional act.
Either way, the patient may feel very anxious and agitated. Allowing him several hours to wash and dress will increase his anxiety and may not help him in any way. Furthermore, the excessive washing may damage his skin and the continual occupancy of the bathroom with soiling of towels etc., may be a great source of annoyance and provocation to the other patients and domestic staff. On the other hand, to restrict him from performing his act will make him frustrated. A choice must be made between the lesser of two evils.

Before preparing a timetable of workable activities, the nursing team should discuss this with the medical and other therapeutic team members. A careful plan must then be worked out and this should be discussed with the patient. The nurse must explain that she will be working with him in trying to help him lead a fuller life by alleviating his anxiety and compulsion to perform his act. The patient will derive security from the knowledge that the nurse is attempting a routine which will enable him to tolerate his tension.

A programme designed for a patient who spends several hours per day washing and dressing may vary but could work as follows:

Phase one	Allow 1 hour for washing and dressing
Phase two	Allow ¾ hour for washing and dressing
Phase three	Allow ½ hour for washing and dressing
Phase four	Allow same time as required by the rest of the ward patients.

At other times the patient should participate in occupational, social and recreational therapies.

14
Hysteria and
Other Neuroses

Hysteria

This is a disorder in which physical or mental disturbance occurs due to an unconscious attempt by the patient to deal with overwhelming conflicts. The patient's symptoms are a compromise or gained advantage in solving some conflict, thereby serving to get him out of some unpleasant situation.

Hysterical personality

While severe stress may produce an hysterical reaction in any person, the symptoms of hysteria are most likely to occur in someone with an hysterical personality.

People with this particular kind of personality are immature and show increased suggestibility, so that they are easily influenced by individuals or ideas that appeal to them. They over-react to situations with a theatrical type of behaviour aimed to impress and gain sympathy. Their reactions to life remain infantile and they cannot adjust at an adult level. They are selfish and preoccupied with their own interests. They crave attention and become annoyed if they do not get it. They are moody and impulsive, and will often go to any lengths to gain attention and sympathy, even to the extent of self-mutilation.

Symptoms

The symptoms of hysteria may be physical or mental or both.

Physical (conversion reactions)

(a) Paralysis of one or more limbs. The paralysis is one of function and not of movement of individual muscles. To the patient, the paralysis is real, and, if it is long-lasting, muscle wasting of the affected part occurs.
(b) Aphonia, or inability to speak above a whisper.
(c) Tremors, tics, spasms, contractures and stammering may also be found.

(d) Sensory disturbance such as anaesthesia, paraesthesia, blindness and deafness may occur.

(e) Visceral symptoms may show as attacks of pain, vomiting, tachycardia, belching, diarrhoea and flatus.

Mental (dissociative reactions)

(a) Amnesia or loss of memory for certain events and people in the patient's life may occur.

(b) A fugue state, or 'twilight' state whereby the patient may wander for hours or days and then find himself in some strange place with no memory as to how he got there, may occur.

(c) Stupors, trance-like states, sleep walking and dual type personalities (e.g. Jekyll and Hyde) are other types of mental disturbances which may be found.

Recognising hysterical convulsions

Some patients may fake convulsions similar to those occurring in epilepsy. However, the following points are familiar to the hysterical convulsion:

(1) Attacks may occur in the presence of onlookers.

(2) The patient does not hurt himself.

(3) He is not completely unconscious and deep reflexes are present.

(4) There is no incontinence, tongue biting or cyanosis.

(5) The well-defined stages of the grand mal epileptic fit are absent. The face becomes red rather than blue.

Causes

The word 'hysteria' was used by the Greeks and means 'wandering of the uterus'. Hysteria occurs in both sexes but is more common in women. The cause may not always be clear but the following may be important:

(a) Early development. Hysterical tendencies are fostered by an over-protective upbringing in childhood. This approach may encourage infantile attitudes and the child may learn to seek attention and dependence by developing ways of manipulating situations for his own ends.

(b) Stress. Hysterical reactions occur more frequently in times of stress (e.g. when experiencing financial problems, marriage difficulties, disappointments and so on).

(c) Injury. Damage to the brain or other part of the body may cause an hysterical reaction. Sometimes the symptoms of physical disease or injury may be unconsciously exaggerated for some psychological gain or where there is an opportunity for financial gain (e.g. compensation).

(d) Heredity. Hereditary, genetic and constitutional factors may be important.

Differential Diagnosis

1. Organic conditions. Early neurological symptoms may be confused with hysteria (e.g. disseminated sclerosis).
2. Anxiety states. Many hysterical patients may complain of anxiety. However, where there is *la belle indifférence* (i.e. the patient is not worried or bothered by his symptoms) an anxiety state can be excluded.
3. Malingering. Hysteria is not to be confused with malingering. The latter is a conscious production of symptoms for gain or for a situation which the person wishes to evade.

Management and treatment

(1) Rest. For Patients with incapacitating symptoms it may be necessary to change the patient's environment and admit him to hospital for rest and treatment.
(2) Drugs. (i) Diazepam (Valium), 6−30 mg orally daily may be given to help relieve anxiety. (ii) Sedation may also be necessary.
(3) Hypnosis (with or without drugs), to relieve symptoms such as aphonia, deafness, amnesia and paralysis.

Nursing care

The physical and psychological symptoms of hysteria occur to solve conflicting situations, and the patient's reactions are often demanding of attention and sympathy. The aim of care and treatment may be designed to discover the patient's conflict and help him to learn a more satisfactory and acceptable way to deal with it. Though the patient's demanding personality may appear off-putting, the nurse must learn to understand his behaviour and give interest, sympathy and attention.

The nurse must persevere in her attempts to convey to the patient how unnecessary it is to maintain the symptoms. The patient must be reassured and helped to discover that there are more rational and acceptable ways to attract attention or gain favours than by hysterical outbursts, self-injury, and other reactions. The nurse must accept and respect the patient and at the same time give him encouragement to solve problems realistically.

Hysterical reactions

Acute reactions such as fits, outbursts, and wrist-slashing, may occur in the ward situation. There is usually some gain to be made from the act and the aim is generally to attract attention and interest. They may commonly occur at certain times such as prior to a ward meeting, during a medical round or at visiting time.

Management

The nurse should:
(1) Remain calm and avoid panic. Go to the patient's aid.
(2) Give reassurance and sympathy. Be firm if necessary.
(3) Reassure the other patients or relatives.
(4) Send for medical help and give first aid if required.
(5) Report the incident and discuss the episode at the next ward staff meeting.

Other neurotic conditions

Reactive depression (exogenous – from without)

Reactive or neurotic depression arises as a result of some definite event. The depression is not very deep-seated and may be temporarily lifted by pleasant company or a change of surroundings. Unlike the psychotic depression, the patient is not retarded and does not express depressive delusions.

As a result of some unhappy event such as a divorce, bereavement or illness, the patient becomes miserably depressed.

Clinical picture

The patient looks miserable and complains of being depressed. He dwells on the painful memories which are making him depressed and he is unable to concentrate on anything else. He is anxious about his physical health and complains of headaches, palpitations, abdominal upsets, constipation, tiredness, lack of energy, insomnia, poor appetite and sexual upsets. In time he recovers completely but may relapse if life treats him badly again. It has been observed that reactive depression is more common in young people.

Management and treatment

Out-patients
Hospitalisation is not necessary for the majority of neurotic depressions. The family doctor will prescribe antidepressant drugs of either the tricyclic variety or the monoamine oxidase inhibitors and sedation to promote a good night's rest. Occasionally the patient's environment may need changing (e.g. a change of occupation).

In hospital
If suicidal tendencies are present, hospitalisation is preferred.
(1) Sedation, rest and observation.
(2) Drugs. Antidepressants e.g. monoamine oxidase inhibitors (MAOI) such as phenelzine (Nardil), 15 mg three times daily. It is stated that MAOI antidepressants are more effective in neurotic depression than tricyclic antidepressants. However, there are exceptions to the rule and tricyclic drugs such as imipramine (Tofranil), 25 mg three times daily, may be used.
(3) Psychotherapy. One-to-one psychotherapy or group therapy may be very helpful.
(4) Electroconvulsive therapy (ECT). This is rarely used but there may be exceptions to the rule.
(5) Recreational and occupational therapy.

Nursing care

The nursing care will be as for a depressed patient and suicidal patient. This is dealt with in detail in chapters 18 and 19.

Compensation neurosis

This neurosis may commonly be seen after industrial accidents and the prospect of receiving money from a compensation claim may be a strong factor in maintaining the condition.

There is frequently physical damage as a result of the accident but following recovery the patient continues to complain and symptoms may be numerous. For example, complaints of throbbing headaches, blackouts, dislike of noise, difficulty in concentrating, insomnia, moodiness, anxiety, giddiness, aches and pains, and inability to work.

The type of person who develops this disease is usually neurotic or with a strong neurotic predisposition. In some instances the injury triggers off conflict or anxiety, and hysterical manifestations may be responsible for the complaining symptoms.

15

Behaviour Modification

Behaviour therapy (*Modification*) describes a group of systematic treatments based directly on the results of experiments on learning theory. Wolpe (1973) defines behaviour therapy as, 'the use of experimentally established principles of learning for the purpose of changing unadaptive behaviour. Unadapted habits are weakened and eliminated: adaptive habits are initiated and strengthened'. The principle of this treatment is that all behaviour is learned and that behaviours, both desirable and undesirable, occur only if they are rewarded (reinforced). A behaviour is explained as those actions of an individual that can be objectively assessed. For example, reporting that a patient is violent is not descriptive but reporting how many times he physically assaulted others is. (See also Bird, Marks and Lindley (1979) in reading list on p. 287).

Behaviour Modification programmes can be planned for an individual or a group. Technique may vary depending on the type of problem. *A Working Party Report*, HMSO (1980), noted two therapeutic approaches. The first emphasises individual treatment mainly for psycho–neurotic behaviour disorders (such as phobias, anxiety, obsessions, sex problems and anorexia nervosa). The second emphasises a group treatment aimed at modifying un-desirable behaviour in the individual through organised group participation chiefly for long stay mentally ill and mentally handicapped (e.g. *undesirable behaviours* such as untidiness, messy eating, uncommunicativeness, destructive behaviour, crazy talk, delusions, etc.).

Behavioural methods are used widely in health care program-mes and may be implemented in various care settings (including the home) by nurses and other health team members. Treatments are planned to meet the individual needs of patients for specified behaviours which the therapist and patient agree needs changing. A big advantage is that the patient participates in solving his own problem. Patients who are treated at home may be helped by their relatives to progress through each stage of a programme.

Techniques

1 **Desensitisation**. This procedure exposes the patient to situ-ations or objects which cause maladaptive behaviour (such as

anxiety, phobias and obsessions). The therapist and patient classify a hierarchy from the least to the most anxiety-provoking situations or objects. A programme is then designed to expose the patient to a controlled sequence of situations which resemble those causing the maladaptive behaviour.

2 Flooding. Desensitisation is a gradual exposure of the patient to situations inducing anxiety or fear. Flooding differs in that the patient is made to confront the situation or object directly. That is, the patient is *exposed in vivo* to the most anxiety-provoking stimulus, from which he cannot escape.

3 Operant Conditioning. This is based on *skinnerian conditioning* (see note B. T. Skinner, p. 103) which stresses the powerful effect which *rewards* have if they are made conditional upon the person's behaviour. Desirable behavioural responses are followed by immediate reinforcement, while undesirable behaviours are punished by withholding the reward. A number of techniques and terminologies is involved as follows:

(a) **Positive Reinforcement**. The patient is given a reward after the desirable behaviour occurs. The aim of the reward is to increase the frequency or improve the quality of the behaviour. Reinforcers may include *social rewards* (such as verbal approval, see Fig. 15.1), *material rewards* (such as food or money) and privileges (such as freedom from ward routines).

(b) **Negative Reinforcement**. This is used to increase the frequency of a specified behaviour by removing the undesirable stimulus after the appropriate response.

(c) **Time Out**. (From positive reinforcement). The patient is removed from a reinforcement session if his behaviour is undesirable. The time out period should not exceed half an hour. Time out is ended when the patient is cooperative or shows signs of exercising desirable behaviour.

(d) **Aversion Stimulation (or therapy)**. A painful or unpleasant stimulus is given upon the occurrence of an undesirable behaviour in the hope that the strength of the habit will be diminished. Aversive stimuli may include electric shock, drugs (in alcoholism) and verbal reprimands from staff.

(e) **Token Economy**. This is an organised reward system often applied to all the individuals in a ward. Everything that happens in the patient's life on the ward can be incorporated into this *motivational system*. Patients are given tokens after each desirable response (positive reinforcement). Tokens are retained by the patient and can be exchanged for goods or luxuries.

B. F. Skinner. An American psychologist and a leading supporter of programmed instruction in which the principles of learning determined on animals in the laboratory are applied to teaching. Skinner is also a behavioural psychologist, that branch of psychology which studies the observable behaviour of man.

Skinner is identified with the concept of instrumental conditioning (i.e. conditioning of a behaviour by reward). Instrumental conditioning differs from Pavlov's classical conditioning which is essentially a form of association, whereby a stimulus becomes a sign or signal for another stimulus.

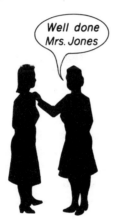

The nurse must be with the patient at each stage and
continually give encouragement and praise achievement

Fig. 15.1 Behaviour programmes

Developing new behaviours

Approaches used in *learning new behaviours* may include:
(i) *Instructions.* The therapist gives verbal or written instructions for the patient to follow (eg how to use a vacuum cleaner).
(ii) *Modelling* (Imitation). This is observational learning in which the patient looks on while the nurse (model) demonstrates the behaviour. For example, the model maintains attention by supplying comments such as 'see how I hold the iron and move it with one hand'.
(iii) *Shaping.* Desirable behaviour is built up in a step-by-step

process. The steps in the shaping process include defining the initial and end *target behaviour*. The total behaviour is then broken down for the patient to learn step by step.

The therapist as a teacher

Helping patients to learn new behaviours (particularly skills) involves the creation of a learning environment, as with the application of all basic teaching principles. Patients need prompting to learn and the behaviour or skill must be motivational in that it can be seen to be of value and relevance. It should also be within the patient's learning capability and reward or satisfaction should be gained from its performance. When teaching a new skill the therapist should:

1 Demonstrate the skill at normal speed.
2 Repeat it at a much slower speed accompanied by a *verbal commentary*.
3 Allow the patient to perform the skill.
4 Encourage the patient to practice until confidence and perfection result.

Learning skills, whether social or motor, can be promoted in an number of ways through discussion, reading, self-help instructions, films or video, learning on the job, role play, *simulation* and *T Groups* — (T-groups consist of about 8 to 12 patients who meet specifically to study the process of interaction in the group itself. The therapist or leader explains that he is there to help them to do this and occasionally intervenes to comment on what is happening).

Planning behavioural care programmes

A systematic framework is necessary to include Assessment → Action Plan → Implementation → Monitoring and Evaluation. It is essentially a *problem orientated approach* and the same principles should apply as outlined in Chapter 11.

Assessment. Initial assessment may be carried out by the doctor and the patient then referred to the *nurse therapist*. Assessment is a critical analytical approach to identify the problem and its susceptibility to a behavioural approach.

Action Plan. A written plan should highlight the actions and roles of both patient and therapist. *Behavioural goals* should be stated and targets set. Particulars about reinforcers or rewards should be included. Criteria for measuring behaviour should be included so that all staff have a standardised approach to reporting.

Implementation. Progress records should be maintained for each patient. Inconsistencies in recording behaviour or allocating rewards should be corrected. Time out periods should be recorded. Tokens allocated should be recorded. At regular intervals the care team should meet for discussion and review of target behaviours and procedures. Patients who are not responding should be reassessed and their programme reviewed to question effectiveness.

Examples of programmes

1 Desensitisation *Problem:* Fear of Swimming
Step 1 Walk to swimming pool.
Step 2 As for 1 plus go inside building. Look at water.
Step 3 Repeat steps 1 and 2. Change into swimsuit. Look at water.
Step 4 As for 3 plus walk a few steps into water.
The hierarchy of steps continue with each one progressing until actual swimming. The therapist supports and reassures at each step.

2 Token Economy *Problem:* Uncommunicativeness

Behaviour	Reinforcer	Timing	Conditional
Talks to therapist	2 Tokens	Each time detected	As part of greeting
Talks to other patients	3 Tokens	Each time detected	As part of interaction.

Guidelines

The *Report of a Joint Working Party* to formulate *ethical guidelines* for the conduct of programmes of *Behaviour Modification*, HMSO (1980), made the following recommendations:
1 Adequate *training* and preparation for staff involved in behaviour modification programme to include in-service training, *multidisciplinary training* and post-basic training.
2 Aims and methods of a behavioural programme should be available to patient and relatives.
3 The patient's or relatives' consent should be obtained. Oral consent is sufficient.
4 *Basic rights* and privileges of patients must be meticulously

respected by all those who design or implement programmes.

5 Where a programme implies restriction of basic privileges this should be temporary and subject to monitoring. Restrictions should be carefully explained to the patient or relative.

6 Responsibilities and authority for programmes should be established and understood by all staff.

7 *A review body* should be established at regional level to monitor behavioural programmes.

8 *Research* into behaviour modification should be encouraged.

References: see Wolpe, J. (1973); Zangwill, O. L. (1980).
Further Reading: see Butler, R. J. and Rosenthall, G. (1978)

16
Schizophrenia

General note on psychotic conditions

The term 'psychoses' refers to those mental disorders in which varying degrees of personality disintegration occur. A psychosis involves change in the whole personality of the subject and is commonly characterised by loss of contact with reality, distortion of perception, regressive (childish) behaviour and attitudes, and abnormal mental content including delusions and hallucinations.

The psychotic patient is less able to act rationally towards the demands of his environment. His thoughts and actions are bizarre and this makes him less able to fit in with the social scene. He looks more untidy and may act in a less inhibited way than the neurotic patient. Outwardly the patient appears grossly abnormal to others but inwardly he appears to be unconcerned about his behaviour or what others think about him. His lack of insight makes it difficult for him to accept treatment or hospitalisation since he cannot realise that he is mentally ill.

Schizophrenia

This is the most common of the psychoses and the biggest cause of disablement among psychiatric patients.

Definition

The term schizophrenia was first used by Bleuler in 1911, and today the term is used to describe what is probably a group of diseases. They are characterised by progressive disintegration or splitting of the mind resulting in:
  (a) disorder of thought and emotion
  (b) loss of drive and withdrawal
  (c) lack of communication
  (d) loss of contact with external reality
  (e) normal behaviour being replaced by abnormal behaviour

Incidence

Between eight and ten people out of every 1000 born today are likely to develop schizophrenia at some time in their lives. Both sexes of all ranges of intelligence are affected. Many never recover fully and almost half the long-stay patients in psychiatric hospitals today have schizophrenia.

Symptoms

Disorder of thought. The person's thinking may be affected in many ways. The association of ideas becomes disconnected and it may be difficult to follow a patient's flow of talk. Thinking may be woolly and the patient never quite gets to the point. Thought blocking as described in previous chapters may occur. Gradually, rational thinking is replaced by fantasy thinking and neologisms (newly constructed words) are formed.

Disorders of emotion. Emotional feeling becomes blunted (flattening of affect) and the patient may appear insensitive and cold. Emotional incongruity or the showing of feelings that are inappropriate to the patient's thoughts or situation occur in many cases.

Loss of drive and will power (volition). The patient loses his drive and ambition. A previously energetic young man may appear lazy by lying in bed until midday and gazing into space instead of working. Dirty habits are a feature of this type, and the appearance is neglected.

Delusions and hallucinations. These, together with ideas of reference, are common. The patient may have delusions of persecution or grandeur and he may hear voices and believe that people are talking about him.

Physical symptoms. In some patients there are abnormalities of thyroid function, and of glucose and nitrogen metabolism.

Clinical types of schizophrenia

Simple schizophrenia

This develops in adolescence or the early twenties. Apathy and lack of emotional response and drive are the most marked features.

The patient fails to live up to earlier expectations of his future. There is a falling off in his standard of work and he may drift from job to job with no clear aims for the future. He may be anti-social and sit around the house all day looking neglected and slovenly in appearance. The patient is dreamy and inattentive; his thinking is woolly and thought blocking occurs.

Hebephrenia

The patient's behaviour is more disturbed and he may be regarded by his friends as odd. Patients with hebephrenia often have outbursts of anger, weeping or grimacing and laughing without adequate reasons, while suicide attempts are not uncommon. Hallucinations of hearing and sight are common and are usually vivid. The patient may have a wild look in his eyes, impulsive behaviour, disjointed speech and inadequate emotional responses.

Eventually the patient may deteriorate and become dirty and incontinent, with impulsive, purposeless behaviour.

Catatonia

This condition is usually acute in onset and takes the form of either stupor or excitement.

When stuporose the patient is inactive and mute. He refuses food, is incontinent and takes no interest in his surroundings. Negativism and waxy flexibility are frequently present. The condition may suddenly change to excitement with impulsive behaviour, hallucinations and aggressive outbursts.

Paranoid schizophrenia (35−45 years)

This type usually occurs in older patients (aged 35−45) and the personality tends to be well preserved for many years. Its chief features are the ideas of reference and delusions of persecution with complete absence of insight and, occasionally, hallucinations.

Note that 'paranoid' describes the feelings of someone who believes that other people are hostile and unfriendly towards him. In some people paranoid traits may predominate in their personality. In many instances delusional paranoid reactions are manifestations of schizophrenia and the terms 'paranoia' and 'paraphrenia' may be used for this type of paranoid schizophrenia.

It is important to note that paranoid delusions may occur in many other conditions. For example, confusional states, alcoholism, depressive illnesses, organic psychotic states and chronic epilepsy.

Chronic schizophrenia

The patient with chronic schizophrenia is usually detached from reality and shows indifference to his activities for daily living. He lives in his abnormal thoughts and ordinary affairs mean little or nothing to him. He behaves very oddly and he may like to dress himself in unusual or bizarre ways. He may be deluded and hallucinated and he may respond to his hallucinations by noisy shouting. The chronic schizophrenic patient usually lacks interest in personal hygiene and appearance and may hoard rubbish. He may talk a language of his own and his conduct may be stereotyped and unpredictable.

Causes

Schizophrenia occurs most frequently between the ages 15–45 years. The condition is rare in children and more common in females than males.

The cause of schizophrenia is unknown. No one factor can be found but it is possible that a number of factors may play a part in its development.

(a) Heredity. It is believed that genetic factors may be a predisposing cause in some people.

(b) Constitution. As previously outlined in Chapter 9, Kretschmer linked the disease with asthenic body build.

(c) Personality. It is estimated that 35 per cent of patients have a pre-psychotic schizoid personality (i.e. quiet, shy, aloof, detached and over-sensitive types who tend to be loners and who day-dream a lot).

(d) Physical factors. Schizophrenia has been linked with endocrine function, physical illness, brain function (EEG irregularities) and biochemical function, but nothing definite is forthcoming from any of these factors.

(e) Psychological factors. Schizophrenia has been linked with faulty early development, conflicts, stress, habit deterioration, and so on.

(f) Social factors. The disease is more common in urban areas than rural areas.

Differential diagnosis

Schizophrenic symptoms may occur in other illnesses, e.g., paranoid reactions in depression and catatonic type states in organic conditions. Toxic-confusion states may occasionally resemble schizophrenia, hysteria and obsessional neurosis.

Management

Out-patients
Some patients may be treated on an out-patient basis. This may involve the family doctor or attendance at a psychiatric out-patient clinic or day hospital.

In hospital
(1) Rest and observation.
(2) Environment. Caring for the patient on a short-term (preferably mixed sex) ward is more stimulating for withdrawal symptoms.
(3) Therapeutic community atmosphere is important, whereby the resources are organised to create a team approach with acceptance of the patient's behaviour and communication (see Chapter 3 on therapeutic community organisation).
(4) Drugs. (i) Trifluoperazine (Stelazine), 2−10 mg three times daily is useful to diminish psychotic behaviour and relieve delusions and hallucinations. Stelazine is more effective for the inert apathetic patient; (ii) chlorpromazine (Largactil), up to 1 g daily also diminishes psychotic symptoms but is more sedative than trifluorperazine (Stelazine). Chlorpromazine (Largactil) is therefore a better drug for the more excited and disturbed patient; (iii) fluphenazine decanoate (Modecate), usually 12.5 mg test dose is given to test susceptibility to extrapyramidal reactions, and then 25 mg every 2−6 weeks. This is a long-acting phenothiazine with similar effects to Stelazine and Largactil. (iv) Other tranquillisers include: promazine (Sparine), thioridazine (Melleril), haloperidol (Serenace) and many others. (v) Anti-Parkinson drugs. Parkinsonian effects are a problem with most of these drugs. Therefore, their administration should be accompanied with drugs such as:
   (a) benzhexol (Artane), start with 1−2 mg daily, then 2−5 mg three times daily;
   (b) orphenadrine (Disipal), 50 mg three times daily;
   (c) benztropine (Cogentin), start with 0.5 mg daily, then 2 mg daily.
(vi) Nitrazepam (Mogadon) may be given for insomnia.
NOTE: Tranquilliser drugs do not cure schizophrenia; they merely keep symptoms controlled and enable the patient to function socially. It is important, therefore, to continue medication for some time.

(5) Electroconvulsive therapy (ECT) may be used to lift stupor or control excitement.

(6) Psychotherapy may have a limited effect but reassurance, persuasion, listening and support are important.

Nursing care

Only a summary of the main points in nursing care will be given here (see below). The nursing care of the schizophrenic patient is so important and varied that it is given specific attention in other chapters to which the reader should refer as follows: ward environment (Chapter 3); behavioural nursing (Chapter 8); withdrawal (Chapter 17); over-activity (Chapter 18); aggression (Chapter 20); institutional neurosis (Chapter 29); dilemma situations (Chapter 36).

The nurse should:

1 Initially, ensure that the patient rests and observe him.

2 Reassure. Many schizophrenic patients are insecure and may be frightened by their feelings and thoughts.

3 Work on relationships. The patient should be encouraged to relate to others, to mix, to communicate and to interest himself in the real world. The relationship may be slow to develop and the patient may not accept or trust the nurse. However, the nurse must persevere and prevent the patient from withdrawing. The nursing relationship can be a potent factor in reinforcing treatment and rehabilitation.

4 Attend to physical care: diet, exercise, sleep, fresh air and weight observation.

5 Persevere and be patient with the patient's odd behaviours. Praise improvements and effort but be firm regarding his personal hygiene and general appearance.

6 Protect the patient during acute episodes, (e.g. absconding, suicide attempts).

7 Manage symptoms as they arise: withdrawal, uncommunicativeness, institutionalism, refusal of food, personal neglect, excitement, stupor, insomnia, delusions, hallucinations and so on.

8 Maintain and develop positive aspects in the patient's personality, e.g. interests, hobbies, family, work and friends, and other contacts outside the hospital.

9 Help friendless patients by introducing them to voluntary workers and others.

10 Remotivate inert and chronic patients.

11 Implement and encourage involvement in recreational, social and work programmes.

12 Administer treatments and note progress, side effects, etc.

13 Prevent deterioration through programmed activities.

14 Maintain dynamism in nursing care by relating with other team members to discuss management and nursing objectives and feedback information.

Rehabilitation

This should start at the moment the patient is admitted and should aim to develop positive aspects of personality and behaviour and maintain links with his family, friends, work and outside world, (relate to Chapter 29). Reality orientation must always be promoted.

After-care

On discharge the patient may require help to find accommodation and work. It may be helpful to involve the patient's friends and relatives more frequently during the later stages of rehabilitation. Also, the social worker and community psychiatric nurses should meet and develop relationships with the patient before he leaves hospital. Consideration should also be given to the role of formal and voluntary agencies in the after-care and an appointment for attendance at the doctor's out-patient clinic should be arranged.

17

The Withdrawn and Unco-operative Patient

1 The withdrawn patient

Patients may withdraw from human contact for a variety of reasons which may include personal, environmental or health factors. The psychiatric nurse will learn to recognise the difference between exaggerated withdrawal occurring as a severe symptom of the patient's illness, and temporary withdrawal occurring as a normal reaction for quiet reflection and relaxation.

Reflecting withdrawal

Some people are by nature quiet and thoughtful. It is part of their personality to withdraw for short periods to create inner quietness, reflect upon thoughts and events, relax, promote peace of mind and plan the resources of their personality. For other patients, there may be occasions when the highly-charged aspects of ward activities and treatment programmes threaten their self-control to such an extent that they feel the need to switch off for a quiet period.

Nursing care

Thoughtful periods of withdrawal are considered to be therapeutic and should be permitted. The assertive nurse who, by the imposition of authority, tries to push quiet patients into contact may cause them to withdraw further and stop communicating. The nurse should learn to recognise the patient's need for quietness as being a normal part of his behaviour. The patient will learn to appreciate the nurse's considerate understanding and this confidence will prove an asset in their relationship.

Exaggerated withdrawal

This type of withdrawal is seen at its most extreme in patients suffering from schizophrenia and in long-stay patients who have spent many years away from human contact. In the former category, the patient is fantasising and out of contact with reality, while in the latter, the patient may consider that he is of no interest to anyone and may feel rejected through having no visitors or individual recognition.

Nursing care

Failure by nursing staff to recognise exaggerated withdrawal can have serious repercussions on the patient's recovery. The nurse should establish a relationship as a basis for promoting contact. This can be difficult but the nurse will learn to time her approaches.

Initially the patient may show anxiety and appear uneasy in the nurse's presence. Sometimes he may reject the nurse but it is important that she does not reject him. The nurse must continue her attempts at contact by returning at regular intervals to the patient. By doing so she is recognising him and showing acceptance. Underneath, the patient may want a closer relationship with the nurse but be afraid of rejection. Once he gets used to the nurse's attention he may be prompted to make overtures which she should recognise, acknowledge and develop.

It is helpful for the nurse to know the patient's interests. Through a knowledge of these, she may be able to appeal for his help and co-operation. At all times she should be aware of activities in which he may take part and encourage him to do so. Once the patient's interests begin to widen, the nurse must encourage him to form friendships and participate in more contact activities. Other staff can become more involved in the patient's contacts, particularly personnel from outside the hospital who often prove very stimulating contacts (for instance, voluntary helpers such as youth organisations and League of Friends).

Opportunity for contact with the opposite sex is important. On occasions, withdrawn patients will make contact with members of the opposite sex but ignore their own sex. A female nurse may achieve more success with a withdrawn male patient and vice versa. More response may be gained by nursing such patients on a ward where there is sex integration. Failing this, every effort should be made to encourage the patient to enter situations which include members of the opposite sex, e.g. patient groups, socials and dances.

2 The unco-operative patient

Patients may be reported as being unco-operative for a variety of reasons which may include refusing medication or meals, refusing to attend therapy, participate in activities or attend to personal hygiene.

The nurse must be objective to avoid reporting a patient as being unco-operative when she really means something else. Also, it is important for the nurse to ask the question 'Why is the patient being unco-operative?' The patient may have some concern about his illness, treatment, or ward environment, which he feels is not being attended to by the staff. Consequently, he may refuse to co-operate in some situation as a means of communicating his plight.

The nurse will learn not to expect the patient's co-operation as a divine right, but rather to develop it as part of her nursing skill. She should rely primarily on her relationship with the patient, but in situations where difficulties are experienced, the practise of skills, and patience in explanation, listening, talking, coaxing and persuasion are essential. It may be more tempting and convenient for the nurse to withdraw from the task and expediently label the patient as being unco-operative; but to do so would be failing in her nursing duty.

Is the patient unco-operative?

Before deciding if the patient is unco-operative, the nurse should ask the following questions:
- Is my request to the patient reasonable?
- Is it necessary for his care or the care of other patients?
- Does the patient understand my request? Have I explained it fully?
- Has the patient been given the opportunity to explain why he is refusing? Have I considered his self-esteem?
- Have I exhausted all my co-operative skills?

If the answer to any of the above is NO, the patient should not be reported as unco-operative.

18

Mania and Depression
(Affective States)

Manic-depressive psychosis

This term refers to a group of illnesses where the patient may suffer recurrent attacks of mania or depression or of both mania and depression.

Individual patients may show a tendency to keep to a definite pattern of breakdowns; some have attacks of depression only, some have mania only and a few may have attacks of both. Indeed, a patient may be labelled manic-depressive even if he has suffered only depressive episodes and never a manic episode.

Causes

(a) Hereditary predisposition. It is estimated that in approximately 11 per cent of patients one or other parent has had the illness.
(b) Pre-psychotic personality. The previous personality may be characterised by either depressive moods (self-absorbed and pessimistic) or elated moods (cheerful and optimistic) or mood swinging (i.e. cyclothymic-swinging from depression to elation).
(c) Pyknic physique. The condition has been linked to people with this body build.
(d) No obvious cause (idiopathic).

Differential diagnosis

Over-activity may also be seen in diseases such as toxic confusional states, schizophrenia, hysteria and excitement due to brain disease, e.g. general paralysis of the insane (GPI).

1 The manic aspect

Suddenly or over a few days the patient becomes over-happy and excited. In the milder degree (hypomania) he is restless, talkative and sleepless. He is bubbling over with enthusiasm and tries to communicate his happiness to others. He may work too hard, trying to do many people's work and taking on too much; he may flit from one thing to another without finishing any and generally be over-confident, boastful and grandiose.

In some cases the condition worsens (acute mania) and the patient becomes obviously ill. He is extremely over-active and noisy. He talks incessantly, jumping from one topic to another (flight of ideas) and he may even shout and sing loudly. He is too excited to eat, drink or sleep and he may become destructive and dirty. In severe cases delirious mania may occur.

At home the manic patient can be a source of great strain on his family, wearing everybody out. In hospital he may be a source of amusement at first, but eventually he becomes an annoyance to the other patients so that great patience and understanding must be engendered by the ward team.

Management and treatment

Exhaustion is always a risk with the manic patient, therefore, the initial treatment will be aimed to promote rest and reduce over-activity.

(1) Drugs which help to reduce excitement and activity include: (i) chlorpromazine (Largactil), 100–200 mg three times daily; (ii) haloperidol (Serenace), 1.5–5 mg three times daily orally; (iii) Lithium carbonate, 400 mg daily is used in some cases and blood checks must be observed to maintain blood lithium levels within 0.6–1.5 mmol/l; (iv) nitrazepam (Mogadon), 5–10 mg at bedtime (night sedation).

(2) Electroconvulsive therapy (ECT) may be used to reduce/ treat the excitement in mania. When used it is given more frequently over a shorter period of time. Careful monitoring and daily review is important.

(3) Psychotherapy is difficult during the acute stage but may be more useful as the patient is recovering.

Nursing care of the over-active patient

Some psychiatric patients are very over-active in the acute stage of their illness. This can be seen at its most extreme in patients suffering from mania but may also arise in alcoholism, drug intoxication, confusion, schizophrenia and following head injuries.

The over-active patient is very restless and may constantly be on the move, he may be excitable and dislike restrictions on his non-stop activity. He may have little time for resting, eating or sleeping, and he may be noisy, untidy and an annoyance to other patients.

Objectives

(1) To reduce activity.
(2) To prevent physical deterioration.
(3) To smooth interpersonal relationships.
(4) To promote rehabilitation.

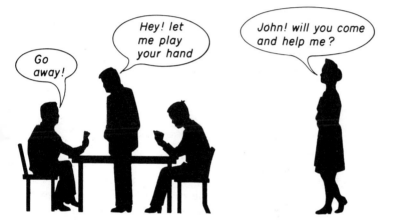

Fig. 18.1 Distracting attention

1 Reducing activity

Sedation will reduce the patient's over-activity but this may take time. During the interval, the nursing staff should prevent the patient from wearing everyone out and exhausting himself. A peaceful, non-stimulating atmosphere should be created and the nursing role required will involve the ability to carry out duties in a quiet, calm and slow manner. The nurse should introduce the patient to activities which reduce his energy and be firm where necessary (especially when he interferes and upsets other patients). Activities which offer outlets for his movements should be encouraged, such as work and physical exercise. The close attention of one nurse may be required in the acute stage of his illness. She should permit freedom to use the ward resources but be prepared to supervise his activity and suggest another if he becomes too involved or makes a nuisance of himself. Over-active patients tend to be easily distracted and the nurse may make a simple suggestion to interrupt him and set him off on something else.

2 Preventing physical deterioration

The patient's neglect of food, fluids, sleep and hygiene endanger his physical health. The nurse should ensure that he attends to his personal hygiene and appearance. He will have little time or enthusiasm for this so a great deal of nursing persuasion and persistence will be needed. The patient may consider eating to be time-wasting but the nurse can encourage him to take sandwiches and food drinks. The patient's excitement prevents him from sleeping and the nurse must promote a sleep-conducive environment to assure rest and prevent exhaustion. A quiet room (free from lights or other distractions), is ideal. There are too many distractions in an open dormitory and his noisy behaviour may keep other patients awake.

3 Promoting interpersonal relationships

The over-active patient's interpersonal skills leave a lot to be desired. Initially, staff and patients may find his company amusing and entertaining but later, even in small doses, he may become annoying and intolerable. He may interfere in other patients' business; constantly interrupt others' conversations; gatecrash discussion groups; fail to keep promises and embarrass visitors. Some patients will accept this behaviour but others may resent it and express hostility towards him. The nurse must distract the patient to keep him from annoying others and if he becomes unbearable, a nurse should stay with him and keep him occupied. It must be remembered that the other patients may have to tolerate his noisy behaviour night and day. The nurse will need to spend some time getting the other patients to understand and accept his behaviour. This can best be achieved in group discussion and at ward meetings.

4 Rehabilitation

As the over-active patient begins to recover, the nurse must help him to become fully accepted again by the other patients. He may be conscious of the embarrassment and upset he has caused and the other patients may still not trust him. The nurse must give him support and encouragement to mix and promote other patients to have confidence in his recovery. He should play a more active part in groups and in recreational, social and occupational activities. The patient's relatives may need reassuring that he is returning to his old self again and prior to discharge they should be informed about aftercare.

2 The depressive aspect

The depressive phase of manic-depressive psychosis may sometimes be referred to as *endogenous depression* and at other times, *psychotic depression*. Again, like the reactive depression already described in Chapter 14, the patient looks and feels miserable. However, this type of depression is more deep-seated and there is a greater degree of hopelessness.

The difference between the clinical pictures seen in psychotic depression and neurotic (reactive) depression can be summarised as follows:

Psychotic Depression	*Neurotic Depression*
The patient's mood shows no response to environmental changes	The mood may lift in cheerful company
Early morning waking occurs	There is difficulty getting off to sleep
Psychomotor retardation is present, thoughts and actions are slow	Only fatigue and tiredness. No retardation present
Depressive delusions are common	Delusions never present

Psychological features

In manic-depression the patient is obviously ill. He may feel that he is a failure in life and that nothing is worth living for. He may feel that he is wicked and that his achievements have been obtained by fraud. He sees no future for himself but despair and hopelessness. His depressive delusions and ideas, along with his other symptoms, may prompt him to end it all by committing suicide. In some cases a depressed person may murder his family or loved one then kill himself. In most cases motor retardation (slow movements and speech) and lack of concentration are present.

Physical features

Constipation, insomnia, loss of appetite and weight, loss of sex drive, headaches, lack of energy, dry mouth and amenorrhoea (in females) are the main physical effects of this depression.

Classification

Endogenous depression may be classified as mild, acute or severe. In severe cases a depressive stupor may feature.

Management and treatment

This is a deep depression which usually requires hospitalisation.
(1) Rest and observation for suicidal tendencies.
(2) Drugs, one selected from an antidepressant group, with a tranquilliser and sedative if necessary.
(a) Tricyclic group antidepressants – (i) imipramine (Tofranil), 25 mg three times daily; (ii) amitriptyline (Tryptizol), 25 mg three times daily; (iii) trimipramine (Surmontil), 25 mg three times daily; (iv) clomipramine (Anafranil), 25 mg three times daily.
Tricyclics should be used with caution in patients with liver disease, epilepsy, or where an anticholinergic drug would worsen the condition, e.g., glaucoma, retention of urine, pregnancy and prostate gland enlargement. Tricyclics affect the actions of other drugs which may be administered at the same time, e.g., alcohol and anti-hypertensives.
(b) Monoamine oxidase inhibitor antidepressants (MAOI's) – (i) phenelzine (Nardil) 15 mg three times daily; (ii) isocarboxazid (Marplan) 10 mg three times daily; (iii) tranylcypromine (Parnate), 10 mg twice to three times daily.
  MAOI antidepressants may potentiate the action of many drugs and foods with sometimes fatal results. Drugs which do not mix well with MAOI's include other antidepressants (tricyclic), barbiturates, alcohol, pethidine, antihistamines and insulin preparations. Food and drink to avoid completely during treatment include: bovril, broad beans, cheese, marmite, yoghurt, oxo and other meat extracts, beer, wines and spirits. These foods interact with MAOI's to cause hypertension.
(c) Tranquillisers may be used to reduce tension and agitation e.g. chlorpromazine or diazepam.
(d) Nitrazepam may be used to promote sleep.
(3) Electroconvulsive therapy (ECT). This treatment gets better results with depression than some other illnesses. It may be the

treatment of choice when suicidal tendencies exist.

(4) Psychotherapy. Supportive reassurance, explanation and suggestion are important to promote recovery and reinforce other treatments.

(5) Occupational and recreational therapy. These are important for helping to draw the patient's mind from his depressive thoughts. The patient's concentration is poor, so a gradual introduction to therapies and other group activities is essential.

Involutional melancholia

This is a particular form of depression occurring at the involutional period, which is taken to be from 40–55 years in women and 50–65 years in men. Involutional melancholia is classified separately from the manic-type psychotic depression because:

(a) It occurs among a definite age group.
(b) The personality of the affected persons differs.
(c) The characteristics and prognosis of the illness differ.
(d) There is agitation and anxiety rather than retardation.

The precise cause of the disease is unknown but an attack may be precipitated by an unexpected illness or an operation. Psychological factors may be important because there are many problems with which one has to come to terms at this period in life. For example, it is a time of failing mental and physical powers, of retirement, of reflections on lost opportunities, loss of power and position, feelings of uselessness, the fear of loneliness and financial hardship, the fear of ill health and so on. Though these psychological doubts about the future may be important, the illness may also occur in people whose future is reasonably assured and who have ample money, work and interests.

Clinical picture

The patient is extremely depressed. He has ideas of unworthiness, misery and hopelessness. He may entertain the most absurd ideas about his body. For example, that he has no brain, he has no stomach or heart, he has no organs at all or that he is riddled with cancer. He may believe that he is unworthy of food and refuse to eat. He may blame his past life for his present state and feel that he should be punished for the sins and crimes he has committed.

Unlike the retarded manic depressive, this patient is anxious and agitated, pacing up and down the ward, wringing his hands and lamenting his fate. With insomnia, anorexia and agitation he may become exhausted. Suicide is also a very serious danger with this patient.

The length of the illness tends to be prolonged if untreated and the prognosis is always more grave than that of manic depression.

Differential diagnosis

1. Hypochondriasis. The patient should not be dismissed as being purely hypochondriacal.
2. Distinguish from other types of depression by noting the age of patient, absence of previous cyclothymic personality and the presence of agitation with delusions of bodily function.
3. Dementia.

Management and treatment

(1) Rest and observation for suicidal tendencies.
(2) Psychotherapy, reassurance and support.
(3) Drugs. (i) **Antidepressant drugs** (as outlined for manic-depression); (ii) chlorpromazine for day time sedation; (iii) nitrazepam for insomnia.
(4) Electroconvulsive therapy (ECT).
(5) Modified insulin therapy to overcome nutritional problems in some cases.
(6) Thorough physical examination to exclude physical disorder.
(7) Occupation and recreation in some form or other. Selectivity is important due to poor concentration.

General notes on depression

In the 1930's the debate existed as to whether there were two types of depression to be called exogenous (caused from without) and endogenous (caused from within) or whether there was only the entity of depression but with varying severity and experienced in different ways by different people. The debate continues with support for both views.

Meanwhile the classification recognises two general groupings which correspond to the clinical concepts of reactive and endogenous depression. Depression may also be clinically named according to other factors. For example, depression in the elderly (senile depression) and depression associated with childbirth (puerperal depression).

From the nurse's viewpoint it is helpful to appreciate that all depressed patients have varying degrees of misery with varying degrees of physical symptoms. The nature and circumstances of the patient's feelings are such that he may attempt suicide and this is a factor which must not be overlooked.

Nursing care

Physical care
The degree of nursing care necessary will depend on the depth of the depression. If the patient is handicapped by stupor or severe retardation to the extent of being unable to look after himself, he may require detailed nursing care. As soon as the depression begins to lift however, mobility must be encouraged. With few exceptions the majority of depressed patients do not require bed care and must be encouraged to be up and about the ward. The nurse should:

1 Encourage and supervise to maintain personal hygiene and appearance, adequate diet and fluids.
2 Promote exercise, fresh air, relaxation and sleep.
3 Prevent pressure sores, mouth infection and constipation.
4 Observe for signs of physical deterioration and prevent self-injury.
5 Administer medicines and observe for drug reactions.

Caring for the patient's physical needs provides the nurse with a good opportunity for forming a relationship. Initially he may be uninterested and non-responsive. Nevertheless, the fact that the nurse is showing interest in the patient (by encouraging him to attend to his needs and, in some cases, by doing things for him) will help him to place trust in her and accept that she cares for him as a person regardless of his own feelings of despair, hopelessness and failure. By caring for his needs she is demonstrating that, as far as she is concerned, his life is worthwhile and his future worth promoting. This will help the patient to understand that all is not lost, as well as building the basis of a good relationship which will help the patient even further when his depression begins to lift.

Psychological care
The nurse will learn to understand the depressed patient. She should relate to her insight of depression: the way it affects the patient's feelings for present existence and future expectations; the way it stagnates his outlook for living and contributing; the way it drains him physically, exhausts him emotionally and so on. By doing so, the nurse learns to accept the patient's behaviour and

appreciate that it is motivated by his melancholic thoughts and feelings.

Remaining with the patient gives him emotional support though outwardly he may not show this by his lack of interest and uncommunicativeness. The nurse should give him her time, attention and sympathy as it reassures him in his basic need for acceptance and approval.

The nurse should take time and sit with the patient when she can. She should listen to him as he talks about his hopelessness and despair as he contemplates each new day, for such a simple approach can be therapeutic. Even if he does not speak, he is aware that she is interested in him and this may renew his hope and confidence.

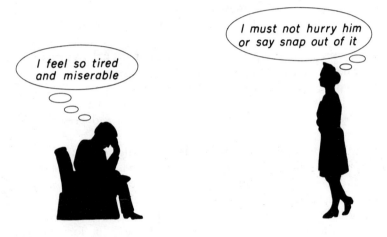

Fig. 18.2 The depressed patient

The patient should be encouraged to take part in activities and to mix with other patients. The nurse should always watch for the slightest sign of interest and develop this further. Initially the patient may appear to have no interest, so when talking to the patient she should discuss things which may be meaningful to him, such as his work, family, children and so on.

Slowly, as the patient begins to improve, he will recognise his thoughts and feelings as part of his illness and thus a different perspective of them will follow. A greater involvement in social and occupational activities can now be introduced. The patient is now more ready for group participation and his recovery will become more enjoyable and satisfying.

Suicidal tendencies

Depressed patients may consider suicide as an acceptable way out of their hopeless, despairing situation. Some make suicide attempts which require casualty treatment and a few succeed in ending their lives. Patients with marked depressive delusions may attempt to harm their families because they believe they should be spared the miseries of this life. And occasionally, mothers with severe depression following childbirth may commit infanticide. Suicide, its management and treatment, will be discussed in more detail in the next chapter.

19
Nursing Suicidal, Deluded and Hallucinated Patients

1 The suicidal patient

Suicidal behaviour may be an attempt to attract attention, to manipulate the environment, or, in extreme cases, to inflict fatal injury. While a large number of people attempt suicide (some more than once), only a small number of these attempts will actually result in death. It is difficult to compile accurate figures on the number of deaths from suicidal behaviour. Some authorities believe that some deaths listed as accidental may actually be suicides. The suicide rate in psychiatric hospitals (England and Wales) is about five times that of the general population. This is equivalent to about one suicide per year in a hospital of 2000 patients, but this figure may be higher for acute psychiatric units and open admission wards.

Why suicidal behaviour?

Incidence

Suicide is included in the first ten causes of adult deaths in industrialised countries (Slater and Roth, 1972). *World Health Organisation Statistics* (1961) showed wide differences in rates between countries. More recent figures issued by the *European Economic Community* (1982) reflect these differences and show Ireland and Britain to have among the lowest suicide rates of the 10 EEC countries (see Table 19.1).

Motivating factors

Widowhood and divorce, separation caused by the death of a loved one, rejection and long term hospitalisation, incurable ill health, old age, bankruptcy, career failure and physical disability are all possible motives behind suicide attempts.

Table 19.1 Suicides per 100 000 of population (figures refer to 1980 unless otherwise stated)

Denmark	31.58	
West Germany	20.90	
France	19.25	
Belgium	19.01	(1977)
Luxemburg	18.08	(1978)
Netherlands	10.09	
Britain	7.71	
Italy	4.62	(1979)
Ireland	3.06	
Greece	2.89	(1979)

Sociological views

Durkheim, in his study *On Suicide* (1897), demonstrates the relationship between suicide rates and the level of integration of individuals into social groups. Highly integrated persons, he argues, are less likely to commit suicide and this may explain why suicide rates are higher among single, elderly, widowed and divorced people.

Durkheim explains three types of suicide as follows:

(a) *Egotistic suicide*. He sees this occurring in persons over whom society has little control, such as the mentally ill and depraved.

(b) *Altruistic suicide*. This type occurs in people over whom society has a strong hold. For example, the aged and chronically sick who may feel a burden on society, and those such as the men who piloted 'suicide' dive bombs for their country during the Second World War.

(c) *Anomic suicide*. This type occurs in persons who find themselves in an insecure social environment due to a disruption of social norms and values. For example, a decline in religious values, relaxation of moral codes or reduced emphasis on the importance of institutions such as marriage.

Psychiatric illness

About one third of those who commit suicide suffer from a serious psychiatric disorder such as:

(a) Depressive illness, hopelessness, guilt and unworthiness.

(b) Schizophrenia, bizarre delusions and hallucinatory voices.

(c) Psychopathic disorder, impulsive behaviour, spite and manipulation.

(d) Hysteria, (attention seeking) and organic degenerative states.

Recognising suicidal behaviour

When caring for psychiatric patients the nurse must observe for behaviour symptoms which may warn her that the patient is contemplating suicide:

(1) Evidence of previous suicidal behaviour or writing suicidal notes.

(2) Depression, lack of communication and early morning waking. Evidence of feelings of guilt and unworthiness.

(3) Hoarding medication or preoccupation with other suicidal hazards.

(4) Talking about death and the futility of living.

(5) Sudden change in behaviour such as restlessness or the appearance of happiness which is masking his real feelings.

(6) Intuition – sometimes the nurse may have an uneasy feeling that something is wrong with the patient but cannot fully identify what it is.

The majority of suicidal patients are managed in the trust and freedom of the open ward. Preventive restrictive measures, (such as supervising medication, bathing and the use of sharp instruments), are necessary but over-protection, restriction and deprivation can be unhealthy and demoralising, not only for the patient concerned, but for the whole ward population.

The formation of a good relationship with the patient can be the most effective preventive measure. It demonstrates to the patient that someone trusts him, cares for him and wants to help. The nurse must give support and encouragement to the patient. She

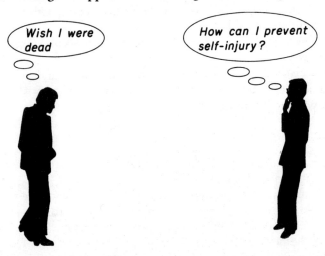

Fig. 19.1 Nursing the suicidal patient

must help him to believe that his life is worthwhile and that others care for him and want him to get well. She must give companionship to the patient and encourage him to come and talk to her if he feels like harming himself. She should cultivate his interests and participate with him in social and occupational activities. She must encourage the patient to talk about his feelings and help him to understand his destructive tendencies. And, above all, the nurse must promote the patient's self-esteem rather than imply through her attitude that he is unreliable and not to be trusted. (See also suicide incident evaluation, Chapter 36.)

Some suicide hazards

The following should be remembered as potentially hazardous to the suicidal patient:
 (a) Bathrooms and toilets
 (b) Power points and electric appliances
 (c) Medications and sharp instruments
 (d) Railways, public highways and waterways

2 Patients with delusions and hallucinations

The nursing problems resulting from delusions and hallucinations are similar.

Some general points

The nurse should NOT:
(1) Argue with the patient over his symptoms. Discuss—Yes. Argue—No.
(2) Reinforce delusions or hallucinations.
(3) Forget that she may be part of the patient's delusional hallucinatory system.
(4) Fail to realise that the symptoms are real to him or to understand his behavioural reactions.
(5) The nurse should try to divert the patient's conversation and attention from his delusions or hallucinations.

1 The suspicious patient

The suspicious patient may be convinced that people are against him: plotting his downfall, belittling his status, trying to poison him and so on. Generally he may be frightened and anxious about his well-being and may be hostile to others for his self-defence. He may find it difficult to trust people because he is not sure if they are acting against him. He may refuse treatment or food and will not mix well. He tends to remain aloof and suspicious, believing that it is safer to remain solitary.

Nursing care

The nursing relationship should aim to maintain a kindly attitude and appeal to the patient's trust. The nurse must prove, through her actions, that she is not against him but understands how he feels. The nurse should not avoid the patient, neither should she make him feel crowded through her probing. Both approaches will increase suspicion. Staff should not whisper in his presence, and gestures (such as pointing out), are likely to cause the patient to feel that he is being singled out.

The patient should not be made to feel restricted by the ward atmosphere. Nursing control may make the patient feel threatened and reinforce his delusions. A liberal programme which allows freedom of choice in his activities and movement must be balanced against the patient's safety and the protection of other patients. Hostility and aggressive urges should be talked out with the patient and directed into ward activities.

The patient's physical health should be maintained. This may be threatened (in some patients) by their refusal to eat 'poisoned food'. The nurse should accept what he says as being real to him and reassure where necessary. It may help (if coaxing and persuasion fail) to allow the patient to participate with staff in preparing his own meal. Sometimes the determined nurse may taste the food from his plate in an attempt to calm his fears.

The patient's developing acceptance of the nurse should help her to increase his trust in other patients and staff. Encouraging the patient to participate in activities may be difficult at first (due to his solitary and suspicious nature) but later, involvement in group activities is necessary to strengthen his trust in others and prepare him for relationships when he leaves hospital.

2 The unworthy patient

Delusions of unworthiness occur most commonly in severely depressed patients. The patient feels inadequate and may believe that he is a failure in life. He may think that he has let down everyone who depended on him and is unfit to live. Some feel inadequate and guilt-ridden and may believe that they would be doing everyone a favour by committing suicide.

Nursing care

The patient is nursed in the overall context of being depressed. Specifically, the nurse must aim to restore the patient's feelings of adequacy and self-confidence. A great deal of reassurance will be needed and he should be encouraged to discuss the positive aspects of his life. The nursing relationship should aim to boost his self-esteem and diminish his feeling of unworthiness. As the patient learns from the nurse he will begin to feel less of a failure. He must be helped to understand that his feelings are a symptom of his illness and are not borne out by his actual achievements in life. He is not a failure, his life is worthwhile, and the friends he believes he let down do not share his pessimism.

3 The grandiose patient

Some patients (e.g., in mania, schizophrenia and general paralysis of the insane), may think they are very important people such as millionaires, prime ministers or royalty. Generally, their be-haviour is not greatly affected by their delusions and they are nursed in the context of the underlying illness. Occasionally, however, the patient may act out the part and behave according to his delusion. For example, the 'millionaire' may purchase expens-ive items he cannot pay for. In such cases, the nurse must help the patient to protect himself from becoming involved in matters which he cannot control. In doing so, there is always a risk that the patient may become annoyed because the nurse is ignoring his importance. Nevertheless, using tact and understanding the relationship should survive such trials.

4 The voices

The patient with auditory hallucinations may claim that he hears voices when it is obvious that no one is talking to him. The voices may threaten the patient causing him to feel frightened and behave unpredictably. The patient will need a great deal of reassurance, help and support. With a calm, quiet approach the nurse should ex-plain what is happening around him, enabling him to distinguish reality from unreality. It is pointless to explain the sensation as being a product of his imagination, to him it is real and meaningful. The nurse should listen and allow him to explain what he hears. She should not agree that she can hear the voice as well, but merely listen and explain. This approach will help the patient to feel better because the nurse is interested in his feelings and experiences. By showing a calm understanding approach she will not reinforce his hallucination and neither will she antagonise him into disagreement or mistrust.

20

The Aggressive Patient

Aggression in society

Aggression is a normal biological potential in each individual. Positively, it is necessary for the survival of the individual and of the species, but negatively, it may cause individual disharmony and even threaten society.

Small children are aggressive when frustrated or anxious. They may express this readily in damage to their toys, temper tantrums and so on. But as they grow into adulthood, they learn to control their aggression and will only express it in a socially acceptable manner. This is not to say that adults are never aggressive – they are. Aggression in society may be fostered by many factors but the following are the most important:

Failure of social controls

During times of war or when there is a breakdown in law and order, people will commit aggressive acts more readily. The Second World War caused man to commit many violent acts and more recently, the collapse of law and order in numerous national conflicts produced similar responses. Removal of restrictions in a psychiatric ward may have a similar effect. For example, neglectful management may cause staff to be less tolerant towards patients and patients towards each other. Violence begets violence.

Frustration

Frustration is a common cause of aggression. For example, in the frustrated mother who batters her baby; or the psychiatric patient whose tolerance breaks due to frustrating ward or hospital management.

Fear and anxiety

The above factors commonly cause aggression in those who feel threatened or insecure. Minority political or religious groups who feel threatened may strike out against the threatening authority. Patients in psychiatric wards who fear for their safety, either mental or physical, may lash out accordingly.

Failure of individual control mechanisms

Mental illness, alcohol and drugs may make a person less capable of exercising control over his aggressive feelings. Patients with brain damage, schizophrenia, mania, epilepsy, psychopathy and mental handicaps may be unable to control their aggressive urges.

Ward environment and aggression

Factors in the ward environment may foster aggression in both staff and patients:

1 Patient population

Two factors are worth consideration. First, over-populated wards are more frustrating, and secondly, wards with a preponderance of disturbed and unpredictable patient types are more likely to produce interpersonal frictions.

2 Staff/patient ratio

Inadequate ward staffing may be a factor. Shortage of nursing staff means the patient will not get the attention he needs so his frustration may increase and anxiety may intensify.

3 Boredom

Failure to initiate sufficient ward activities may result in patient boredom. Opportunities should be available to promote outlets for excess energies.

4 Communications

Lack of recognised communication outlets for patients and staff are important factors. Patients need opportunities to discuss their problems and staff require open discussion to prevent mis-understandings or inadequate implementation of treatment programmes.

5 Attitudes

Staff attitudes may contribute to aggressive behaviour in patients. Ineffective relationships, bossiness, abruptness, disrespect and tactlessness, may prove provocative to some patients.

Recognition and management of aggression

1 Passive aggression

Not all patients present the 'picture' of an aggressive person. Some may suppress their anger and shy away from actions which may be seen as aggressive. Such patients may be aware of their aggression but fear losing control. Instead they may express their feelings by showing anxiety and passivity.

2 Verbal aggression

Patients may become verbally aggressive when they feel frustrated, angry or upset. Reactions may include swearing, shouting or making threatening remarks to staff, visitors or other patients.

Management

Over-zealous intervention to control a verbally aggressive patient may provoke a physical outburst. The nurse should adopt a quiet manner to calm and reassure the patient. The best approach is to allow expression and ignore abuse. When the patient is calm he should be encouraged to talk out his problem and discuss the aggravating factor. Situations where patients use threats to bully other patients are a different matter. This calls for the nurse to calmly, but firmly, divert the bully and reassure the patient who is threatened.

3 Physical aggression

Occasionally some patients may direct their hostility towards persons or property. They may break furniture, smash windows, throw objects, pull hair, tear clothing, scratch or aim blows.

Management

Violent outbursts should be managed in a practical way. Nursing intervention must aim to calm the aggressor and prevent damage to property and injury to person. Intervention will vary depending on the individual patient, the type of outburst and the problems developing from the incident. The hospital's policy for the management of violent outbursts should be consulted.

1 Initial intervention. The situation should be assessed before reacting. It may be possible to placate the patient and direct him away from the object of his aggression by talk and reassurance. The worst possible intervention is nursing over-reaction. The appearance of three or four nurses may cause the patient to feel more threatened and provoke intense resistance. He may be regretting his outburst and needing an opportunity to save face. A one-to-one approach controls most aggressive outbursts.

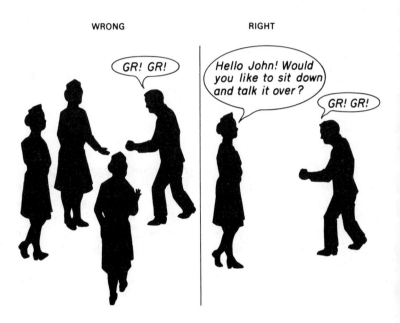

Fig. 20.1   The nurse should avoid over-reacting

2 Restraint. Restraining a patient should be used as a last resort or if the risk of injury is so great as to demand urgent intervention. Restraint may also occasionally be used to administer a prescribed treatment to a resistive patient.

Some patients can be quietly restrained by one nurse grasping her arms around the patient's upper limbs and body from the side position. In situations such as 'hair-pulling' or 'tie-pulling' the nurse should firmly grasp the aggressor's wrists and move towards the patient in order to neutralise the pulling force.

Assessments which conclude that there is a risk of injury to the patient or nurse in a one-to-one struggle, require a team approach.

A minimum of three will be required. With a co-ordinated movement two nurses will grasp simultaneously the upper limbs and body from the side position while the remaining nurse grasps her arms firmly around the patient's lower limbs. The patient may be lowered on to a chair or bed until he becomes calm. A blanket or the patient's jacket may be used to assist restraint. The doctor should be contacted and a sedative injection may be prescribed to further calm the patient and promote 'sleeping it off'. Before leaving the bedroom, nurses should remove objects which may be used as 'missiles'. Throughout the restraint procedure, the patient's dignity and privacy should be protected. He should be observed until he regains composure.

3 Post-violence. The aggressive patient must be helped to recover from the incident and 'climb-down' without loss of face or fear of recrimination. The nurse must reassure the patient and show by her actions that the incident has not effected her relationship with him.

An objective report of the incident should be made. The situation must not be dramatised out of proportion but recorded as part of the patient's progress. If any injuries occur to patient or staff, an accident form must be completed.

Following the incident an effort must be made to discover why the outburst occurred and whether it could have been prevented. A team meeting will be necessary to discuss and analyse critically the evaluation.

4 Incident evaluation. To promote learning and development of management and preventive techniques, the ward team should evaluate each aggressive incident. An interview with the patient should be part of the evaluation process. The following points should be considered:

(1) Does the patient have a history of violent outbursts?
(2) How frequently do outbursts occur?
(3) Is there a pattern to the outbursts (e.g. following therapy, duty shifts, etc.)?
(4) What is the patient's diagnosis and treatment?
(5) Are outbursts related to alteration in illness or mood?
(6) Where do incidents usually take place?
(7) How does he behave in the days/hours proceeding the outburst?
(8) Does he have any other aggressive habits (e.g. temper tantrums, 'bullying', etc)?

(9) Does he have any self-destructive tendencies (self-injury, drug or alcohol abuse)?

(10) What were the patient's feelings before and after the outburst?

(11) Does he show remorse or guilt following the outburst?

(12) How was the incident managed?

(13) If restraint was necessary, how many staff were involved?

(14) How was the patient managed in the hours/days following the incident?

(15) How does the patient feel about the way he was managed?

(16) Were there any injuries to staff/patients or damage to property?

(17) What was the staff/patient ratio at the time of the incident?

Preventing aggression

Consider:
- Ward population and patient content
- Staff/patient ratio
- Interpersonal relationships and staff attitudes
- Treatment and nursing policies
- Communications
- Morale and staff training

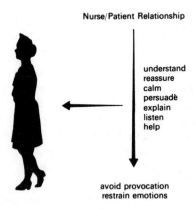

Fig. 20.2   Managing outbursts

21

Psychopathic Disorder and Crime

Psychopathic disorder

The psychopathic person develops as an adult, in the physical sense, but his emotional development and personality show marked immaturity. Psychopaths may be of any intelligence level and some exhibit aggressive tendencies. Though some can be charming and likeable, they have no loyalties to any person, group or code, and neither can they benefit from experience or punishment.

Legal definition

The Mental Health Act for England and Wales, 1983, defines psychopathic disorder as being 'a persistent disorder or disability of mind, (whether or not including significant impairment of intelligence), which results in abnormally aggressive or seriously irresponsible conduct on the part of the person concerned'.

The Butler Committee (1975) recommended that the term psychopathic disorder should be replaced by personality disorder. However, the 1983 Act retains the term.

Features of a psychopath (sociopath)

The features of a psychopathic person may bring him into conflict with society. Common features include:

(1) Anti-social and anti-authority attitudes, irresponsibility, poor judgement.

(2) Emotional immaturity, superficial charm, selfishness and impulsiveness.

(3) Lack of remorse, pathological lying, disloyalty and unreliability.

(4) Ineffectiveness in relationships, unfaithfulness and inability to show affection.

(5) Exhibitionism, dishonesty, demanding behaviour, manipulativeness and immorality.

Incidence

The incidence of psychopathic personality in the population as a whole is 0.25 per cent but the proportion found among the prison population is estimated at 5 per cent.

Causes

The cause is not known but the following factors may be important:
(a) Hereditary, constitutional and environmental factors.
(b) Faulty childhood, e.g. broken home, maternal deprivation, insecurity, poor parental interest and lack of affection.
(c) Brain damage.

Differential diagnosis

It is important to distinguish between episodic psychopathic behaviour as opposed to persistent psychopathic personality.

Clinical types

The intelligent psychopath lives on his wits, has expensive tastes and does not like to work. He may 'con', 'sponge', blackmail, steal and forge cheques. He tends to be charming, well dressed, well spoken and may boast a pseudo-pedigree background. He is a pathological liar and will tend to let down those who trust him. Women may find him fascinating and he will use this to his advantage. Some have vivid sexual fantasies and may commit sexual offences.

The inadequate psychopath lives at a lower level. He is most likely to be one of life's failures as he is unstable, weak-willed, and lacks will power and determination. He shows little restraint and is immature and shallow in his emotions.

The aggressive psychopath has uncontrolled explosive outbursts of aggressive and anti-social behaviour. He can be cold and ruthless and may bully those who are weaker than himself. He shows no guilt or shame for his actions.

Care and management

There is no specific right or wrong approach for treating a person displaying psychopathic tendencies. Some believe in using disipline while others favour a liberal regime. Psychopathic people may be found in a variety of settings. For example, open psychiatric wards, psychopathic treatment centres, security units, special security hospitals, prisons and the community.

Nursing relationship

Nurses may experience different feelings towards psychopathic patients. Some for example may find them to be charming and flattering while others may be disgusted by their immorality, lack of responsibility and lying. Regardless of what their own feelings may be, it is important that they treat each patient as an individual who is entitled to no more, nor less, than any other patient.

It is important that the nurse understands the patient and accepts him for what he is. The patient's past experiences may have convinced him that everyone is for themselves in this world. He may have been starved of love and affection in the past and now feel that his behaviour is essential for survival. He may be convinced that everyone has a price and it is only a matter of paying it, (through flattery, bribery, bullying etc.), to get what he wants.

The nursing relationship must aim at altering the psychopath's behaviour. Occasionally the patient may make trouble for the nurse and exploit other patients. Nevertheless, he must be encouraged to behave responsibly and be given proof that his antics will not work with the ward team. The whole tone of care should be aimed at helping the patient to face his problems and learn that there are other ways to cope with life besides immature behaviour.

Some specific care systems

1 The psychiatric ward

Many psychopathic patients are cared for in the psychiatric wards of ordinary mental hospitals. In the majority of cases a therapeutic approach is used (including group therapy and psychotherapy). The patient is encouraged to mix in situations which will develop his interpersonal relationships. He is encouraged to discuss his feelings and problems. He is given responsibility and helped to understand the effect of his behaviour on others and he is introduced to situations which help him to deal with his problems in a mature and responsible way.

In caring for the psychopathic patient the 'authority bit' should be kept at a low key otherwise the nurse may be re-enforcing the 'them and us' behaviour. This does not mean, however, that the patient should do as he likes. There may be occasions when the nurse will have to be firm by insisting that he follows the treatment and care plan. The balance between permissiveness and firmness in the relationship may be difficult to maintain at times but it is important that this is sustained. Where difficulties are experienced, it is advisable for the nurse to seek advice and perhaps discuss the problem openly at a team meeting. Behaviour modification may help with some problems.

Drug therapy

Drugs are of little value except as a temporary measure. Tranquillisers may help control aggressive behaviour and sexual outbursts may be controlled by hormonal therapy.

2 The Henderson Therapeutic Approach

This approach was started by Dr. Maxwell Jones in 1947, at the Belmont Social Rehabilitation Unit, Surrey. Now known as The Henderson Unit, it practises a system of care which makes the patient responsible for his own actions. Group therapy is used and the patients are encouraged to carry out responsible community tasks. They learn to experience how their behaviour affects society by having a 'taste of their own medicine'. For perhaps the first time in his life, the psychopath becomes both the authority and the victim and the 'they and I' excuse is no longer tolerated.

3 The special hospital system

In England and Scotland, special security hospitals such as Moss Side at Liverpool, Rampton at Nottingham, Broadmoor in Berkshire and Carstairs in Lanarkshire, treat psychopaths with dangerous or criminal tendencies. These hospitals were established to treat only compulsorily detained patients. In terms of administration, special hospitals are identified with the medical system rather than the prison system but the treatment offered is very much determined by security needs. Nursing staff are skilled and concentrate on developing close relationships with the patients but they are authoritarian in terms of supervision, checking, locking doors, counting heads and so on.

4 The prison hospital system

Some prisons have developed hospital wards for psychiatric inmates (mostly psychopaths). For example, Parkhurst Prison, Isle of Wight, has about 35 hospital beds. When in hospital, the prisoners are treated as patients and a therapeutic approach is used.

Crime and mental disorder (forensic psychiatry)

Sometimes a mentally disordered person may commit a crime because he is emotionally disturbed or does not realise what he is doing. Such behaviour is found only in the minority however, and does not imply that most mentally disordered persons are criminals. The following crimes may apply:

Shoplifting

A mentally disordered person with extreme anxiety, depression, forgetfulness, or confusion, may pick up goods in a store without paying for them. Kleptomania is a psychiatric condition whereby the person persistently steals goods which usually he does not need and for which he can well afford to pay.

Physical assault

Some mentally disordered persons may assault other people usually without preplanning. A paranoid patient may attack people he imagines are persecuting him, while a manic or mentally handicapped person may lash out at others in frustration.

Sexual offences

Rape and other sadistic sexual attacks may occur in some psychopathic states. Occasionally sexual attacks may be directed toward children, (Paedophilia).

Arson

The incidence of arson is rising in England and Wales and it is believed that nearly one-fifth of fire insurance claims are for property damaged by arsonist fires. Many arsonists are children from disturbed home backgrounds but occasionally a psychopathic or psychotic-orientated person may become a fire-raiser.

Management and treatment of criminal behaviour

(1) Some unrecognised cases may be dealt with by the courts and either put on probation, fined or sent to prison.

(2) Minor offence patients may enter hospitals informally for psychiatric treatment. In some cases a court order may be used to enforce treatment.

(3) Serious offence criminals are usually detained in a security hospital for treatment.

Secure units

The need for *secure units* developed from difficulties in trying to manage violent, unpredictable or offender patients in the open psychiatric hospital. In 1977, in response to the Butler Report (1975), the Government requested regional health authorities to start building regional secure psychiatric units, consisting of secure in-patient places, out-patient and day treatment facilities for mentally abnormal offenders. These units would be centres of training for many disciplines from the community and prison services as well as the NHS and through their links with hospitals and prisons they would provide better through care with subsequent benefit to the offender.

Meanwhile, many hospitals have designated a ward as an *interim secure environment*. Examples of such units are the Special Assessment and Supervisory Social ward at Cane Hill Hospital, Surrey and the interim secure ward at Prestwich Hospital, Manchester. These wards are locked for security reasons but care programmes are therapeutic with emphasis on individual care, behaviour modification, interpersonal skills and rehabilitation. A six week specialist Post-Basic Clinical Studies Course, No. 960 'Principles of Psychiatric Nursing within Secure Environments', is held at the Royal Bethlem and Maudsley Hospital to prepare staff wishing to specialise in the care of patients exhibiting unpredictable, violent or antisocial behaviours.

22

Alcoholism and Drug Dependence

Alcoholism

The World Health Organisation defines alcoholics as 'those excessive drinkers whose dependence on alcohol has attained such a degree that they show noticeable mental disturbance or an interference with their mental and bodily health, their interpersonal relations and their smooth social economic functioning, or who show the prodromal signs of such developments. They therefore require treatment'.

Stages in dependence

The potential dependent may be a popular young person who enjoys drinking with others and is rarely troubled by hangovers. Gradually his consumption may increase far beyond what is socially acceptable and he may begin to crave alcohol. Many young people presenting themselves to treatment units have reached this level and seek help to give it up.

If unable to overcome their dependence they tend to drift on drinking and their problems mount. In later years their tolerance for alcohol decreases and they become drunk more easily. Their slide down the social ladder continues. They are an employment risk; become unreliable, and their family life may be threatened. Memory disturbance, tremors, blackouts and sleep disturbance occur.

If they continue drinking, more serious deterioration becomes evident. Their social and personal habits deteriorate; they lose self-control and some may begin to live rough. In chronic cases paranoid traits develop in their personality. Unless they give up drinking, serious mental and physical complications will supervene, e.g., delirium tremens, Korsakov's psychosis, cirrhosis of the liver, peripheral neuritis and depression.

Predisposing factors to alcoholism

(a) Parental alcoholism and social learning.
(b) Occupational drinking (e.g. people in the trade).
(c) Loneliness, shyness and inadequate personality.

(d) Mental illness e.g. depression, pre-senile dementia and psychopathy.
(e) Marital disharmony, sexual problems and stress.
(f) Heredity factors and constitution.

Incidence

Alcoholism occurs at all levels in the community and in all intelligence levels. It is more common in men than women and is a problem in the young as well as the old. It is estimated that there are approximately half a million alcoholics in England and Wales.

Complications

Delirium tremens (the horrors)

This is a serious illness which usually follows a few days of abstinence. The patient presents with confusion, restlessness, hallucinations (often visual and frightening), illusions, sweating, insomnia, aggressiveness, loss of appetite and trembling. Pneumonia or injury may intervene and death may result in serious cases.

Cause

Sudden withdrawal of alcohol. Other contributory factors are infection, head injury and poor nutrition.

Management

(1) Bed rest and observation.
(2) Sedation with tranquillisers.
(3) Vitamin B therapy: daily injections of high potency Parentrovite for 7–10 days, followed by oral vitamin B_1 for several weeks. Alcohol interferes with the absorption of vitamin B causing a deficiency which can be counteracted by this treatment.

Nursing care

Nursing care should be planned to fit the individual case following a detailed nursing assessment.
1 Full nursing care (diet, fluids, personal hygiene and pressure areas).

2 Observation and reassurance.
3 Prevention of injury and reduction of confusion (see Chapter 24).
4 TPR chart and intake and output records.

Korsakov's Syndrome

This condition usually occurs as a complication of chronic alcoholism and is thought to be due to the effects on the cerebrum of long standing vitamin deficiency. The disease is characterised by loss of memory, confabulation and disorientation in time. Muscular weakness is also present and peripheral neuritis may be an additional complication. The prognosis is usually poor.

Nursing emphasis should be on reducing confusion, establishing orientation and physical care.

Alcoholic Hallucinosis

The condition occurs as a complication of chronic alcoholism and the main features are hallucinations and delusions of persecution. The course of the disease generally ends either in recovery or dementia. Treatment consists of withdrawal from alcohol, vitamin therapy and chlorpromazine.

Chronic alcoholism

Chronic alcoholism develops when the individual is rarely sober and can no longer control his drinking even though his physical and mental health are impaired.

Mental dysfunction is shown by carelessness, emotional disturbance, unreliability, loss of memory, depression and paranoid ideas. Physical deterioration is usually evident through conditions such as obesity, peptic ulcer, gastritis, chronic bronchitis, cirrhosis of the liver and heart failure. If the patient does not give up alcohol, recovery is unlikely and death will occur due to physical deterioration.

Treatment and care

The treatment for the alcohol dependent will commence with either sudden or gradual withdrawal from alcohol (see also Chapter 35). Drugs such as chlormethiazole (Heminevrin) or chlordiazepoxide (Librium) may be used to combat withdrawal effects and vitamin deficiency may be corrected by injections of Parentrovite. During the initial drying out period the patient will be encouraged to rest, relax, and restore his physical condition. Assessment for follow-up treatment will take place and any acute symptoms, such as delirium, excitement and dehydration, will be treated.

Follow-up treatment. The follow-up treatment will depend on the results of the assessment and the patient's motivation to give up drinking.

Chemotherapy

(i) *Apomorphine.* This is an emetic drug which is given at the same time as a drink of alcohol. The procedure is repeated every two hours. The result is a sorry mess with the patient drinking and being violently sick. The aim of this treatment is to build up an aversion to alcohol and is known as aversion therapy.

(ii) *Antabuse.* When the patient is given Antabuse followed by a drink of alcohol he will experience very unpleasant effects such as breathlessness, choking, palpitations, severe headache and flushing. In some extreme cases he may vomit or collapse. This is known as an Antabuse reaction experience and is conducted under strict medical and nursing supervision. Once the patient has had the experience he is prescribed a daily dose of Antabuse with the knowledge that if he drinks he will be very sick.

Procedure for disulfiram (Antabuse) reaction. Commencing four days prior to the Antabuse reaction experience the patient is given 800 mg disulfiram daily. On the day of the test the patient is given 50 ml of his favourite drink of alcohol. If no reaction occurs after 15 minutes the dose of alcohol is repeated every 20 minutes up to a total period of 1 hour.

Management

(1) Continuous observation and monitoring.
(2) Record pulse rate every 10 mins.
(3) Record B/P every 20 mins.
(4) Continue supervision and observation until reaction reaches climax.
(5) If reaction is not reached, continue supervision and observation as climax may be delayed even to sometime during the night.

Antabuse implant. Alcohol dependents who will not persist with oral disulfiram (Antabuse) may volunteer for the implantation of sterile pellets of Antabuse into the abdominal wall. The operation for implantation takes place some days after the test experience. A 3 cm incision is made and 10 × 100 mg pellets of pure sterilised disulfiram are placed deep in the external oblique muscle of the abdomen. The sutures are removed one week later. Observers following the operation should be on the lookout for possible infection or discharge of pellets from the wound.

Group therapy

Group therapy is now an essential part of many treatment programmes for the alcohol dependent. If the patient's assessment results indicate a motivation to give up drinking, he is referred to the therapy unit. The purpose of the group is to help the patient to come to terms with his problem in a setting with other alcoholics who are striving to do the same. By mixing and discussing with his own dependent colleagues he can learn to see his own behaviour as reflected by others. His fellow patients will also reinforce his motivation.

The actual functioning of each group may differ from one unit to another (see the discussion of group therapy in Chapter 35).

Alcoholics Anonymous (AA)

AA groups are now well developed in most large towns and cities. During treatment the patient will be introduced to AA and encouraged to attend their meetings on leaving hospital. Members of AA meet regularly to discuss experiences and problems. They set a belief that the dependent can overcome his trouble only by surrender and acceptance of some power greater than himself. The dependent must begin by admitting to himself that he is an alcoholic. AA members also work actively in the conversion of other alcoholics.

Al-anon is a group that came into existence for the benefit of the alcoholic's family. It is important to involve the patient's spouse and family in the treatment, and family counselling may be necessary.

Drug dependence

Definition

The World Health Organisation defines drug dependence as 'a state arising from repeated administration of a drug on a periodic or continuous basis'. Its characteristics will vary with the agent involved, but it is a general term selected for its applicability to all types of drug abuse and carries no connotation in regard to degree of risk to public health or need for a particular type of control.

Causes

(a) Many dependents have inadequate personalities and are unable to cope with everyday stresses.
(b) Some may become dependent on drugs prescribed to treat some other condition.
(c) Some get into drugs by chance and contact with other addicts.
(d) Young people may take drugs for 'kicks' or in rebellion against authority.

Drug effects

(i) *Pethidine* – excessive use causes delusions and hallucinations and if suddenly stopped the dependent has attacks of vomiting, diarrhoea, shivering, cramps and convulsions.
(ii) *Morphine* produces euphoria; dependents have pin-point pupils, constipation and sexual impotence. Withdrawal symptoms are similar to pethidine.
(iii) *Heroin* creates a feeling of alertness and increased energy. Pin-point pupils are also present. Generally the dependent looks ill and some may become psychotic or delirious. Withdrawal effects are similar to pethidine but the patient is also more anxious and craves for the drug.
(iv) *Amphetamines* – addiction may follow their use to treat obesity. These drugs increase energy, produce euphoria and promote self-confidence. They may be used by night workers to keep awake. Amphetamine psychosis with hallucinations and paranoid delusions may occur. Withdrawal symptoms do not occur when amphetamines are stopped but depression can be a problem.
(v) *Barbiturates* have a cumulative effect and are a more common addiction than has been realised. They produce anxiety, slurred speech, ataxia, confusion and tremor. The withdrawal effects include sweating, insomnia, irritability, tremor and convulsions.
(vi) *Marihuana* (also known as pot, hashish, cannabis and Indian hemp) produces vivid imagination, frenzy and euphoria. Withdrawal effects are minimal and it is not itself addictive but may lead to taking hard drugs.

Complications

The patient may lose weight and his physical health may deteriorate. He may develop septicaemia, abscesses, hepatitis, or pneumonia. In severe cases death may result.

Treatment and nursing care

1 **Withdrawing the drug.** Withdrawal of the drug is usually carried out in a hospital or treatment unit under strict medical and nursing supervision. Initially the patient will be reassured that everything possible will be done to ease the withdrawal symptoms. Symptoms may vary but generally they may include: trembling, lack of concentration, agitation, anxiety, yawning, tears, sweating, loss of appetite, insomnia, vomiting, diarrhoea, abdominal cramps and fits.

The usual method of withdrawal used is by slowly reducing the dose (weaning off). In all cases the object is to reduce the dose quickly but comfortably. Tranquillisers such as chlorpromazine (Largactil), chlordiazepoxide (Librium) and diazepam (Valium) may be given to ease withdrawal effects. In very selective cases the patient may be allowed to sleep through the withdrawal period using continuous narcosis technique. Withdrawing barbiturates produces a greater risk of fits occuring and the use of phenothiazine tranquillisers are avoided because they tend to add to the risk.

2 **Physical care and rehabilitation.** Initially the patient may require physical care due to his neglect of health during the acute addiction. During this period a relationship should be developed which will be constructive to the patient's attempt to learn a new way of life free from drugs. The nurse's attitude towards the dependent should be one of acceptance and tolerance but she should also be aware of the danger of relapse and the likelihood of drugs being smuggled into the ward.

Rehabilitation is the most important part of the post-withdrawal care. Two major objectives need to be considered:

(a) *Encouraging abstention.* Helping the patient to prepare for a drug-free life begins as soon as withdrawal is complete. The care programme should be designed to help the dependent to develop convincing reasons for giving up drugs. Occasionally this can prove difficult because the dependent is reluctant to face his personal problems and difficulties without the barrier of drugs.

Group therapy, similar to that outlined for alcoholism, is widely used. In the group the dependent mixes with other addicts and is given the opportunity to see his own problems reflected in the other members' behaviour. All the group members have dependence in common and can discuss and share experiences, thus helping each other to recover.

(b) *Long-term rehabilitation.* Although the addict may have lost contact with his family it is important that the social worker re-establishes this. The parents must learn to understand the patient's problem and give support to him when he leaves the treatment unit. The dependent may be poorly motivated and he will need guidance and help to find regular employment. The patient's circle of friends outside hospital may include persons who are still using drugs, consequently, it will be advisable for him to avoid these friendships and also previous haunts where drug-taking is encouraged.

Lastly, before leaving hospital the dependent should be introduced to the local ex-addicts association, providing one exists. This association (known as Synanon) is similar to AA. They hold regular meetings and the ex-addict is helped in rehabilitation. Unfortunately, this association is not wide-spread as AA, therefore the role of the social worker and the out-patient clinic follow-up is very important. The prognosis will depend on how well motivated the dependent is to give up drugs. The community psychiatric nurse has an important supportive role to play in after care. *Drug clinics*, such as Cokehole Trust (Andover, Hampshire), and in London Phoenix House (Forest Hill), Elizabeth House (Earls Court) and City Roads Crisis Intervention Centre (City Road, E.9), are key developments in the care of drug dependents.

Alcoholism and Drug Dependence—a combined approach

A World Health Organisation Expert Committee (1967) in a report (*Services for the Prevention and Treatment of Dependence on Alcohol and other Drugs*) recommended to member nations that alcoholism and other drug dependence should, in spite of certain important differences, be dealt with as basically one problem. This so called combined approach has since been adopted in some treatment units. The concept of joint alcohol and drug dependence treatment units (*ADD units*) set in the context of the district general hospital and supporting community services has been suggested as an ideal way forward in a King Edward's Hospital Fund publication '*Alcohol and Drug Dependence— Treatment and Rehabilitation*' (1972).

23
Diseases of the
Nervous System

A number of conditions which may feature confusion, impairment of memory, orientation judgement and intellect may be due to illness caused by or associated with impairment of brain tissue function. These conditions may be caused by injury to the brain, various physical diseases or toxic conditions.

Core problems

Signs and symptoms will vary with the specific organic conditions but some general problems exist with most syndromes as follows:
1 Personality changes
2 Emotional instability
3 Personal habit deterioration
4 Confusion and irritability
5 Poor concentration and judgement
6 Memory disturbance
7 Loss of interests
8 Wandering and accident risks
9 Physical complications (such as incontinence)
10 Insomnia

Pre-senile dementias

These are degenerative brain diseases which produce dementia and occur before the age of 65 years. Included are Huntington's chorea, Alzheimer's disease and Pick's disease.

Huntington's chorea

1 This is transmitted by a single dominant gene. Fifty per cent of the children of an affected person will develop the condition. It usually runs a course of 10−20 years (the average is 14 years).
2 The onset occurs between 20 to 25 years and produces atrophy of the frontal lobes and basal ganglia.
3 Early manifestations are emotional (e.g. depression and explosive outbursts, sucidal tendencies).

4 Jerky, non-purposeful, involuntary movements of the limbs are a feature. They affect all muscle groups in the face, limbs and trunk.

5 Speech has a staccato quality, like a machine gun. There is apathy, muddled thinking and difficulty in walking and eating.

Management and treatment

There is no cure for Huntington's chorea; symptomatic treatment is used such as:

(1) Tranquillisers and antidepressants as required.

(2) Drugs. Chlordiazepoxide or diazepam may give some relief from the incessant muscular over-activity. Tetrabenazine is a neuroleptic drug and it may be used by some doctors.

(3) Family support – the patient may not need hospitalisation until the disease is well advanced. Social services, family doctor, district nurses and other care agents are very important in the pre-hospital treatment and management.

(4) Occupation and recreation.

(5) Genetic counselling—aims to provide information concerning the nature of the abnormality and to explain the risks an individual has of being affected or of a couple having affected children.

Nursing care is discussed later in this chapter on page 165.

Alzheimer's disease

This form of pre-senile dementia was first described in 1907 by Alzheimer. There is a general atrophy of the brain due to death and degeneration of nerve cells. The atrophy particularly affects the frontal and temporal lobes. The prognosis is very poor.

1 The cause is unknown. It usually runs a course of 5–15 years (average 12).

2 It has general features of dementia as outlined. Periodic insight may occur.

3 Memory loss and disorientation are particularly marked. Dysphasia and apraxia signs are considerable.

4 Mild signs of upper motor neurone involvement show through facial muscle weakness, shuffling gait and slow awkward movement.

5 Fluctuating depression with suicidal tendencies. Fits occur in 30 per cent of cases.

Management and treatment

(1) The patient is cared for at home for as long as possible. Attention should be given to nutrition and exercise.

(2) Social agencies should be mobilised to support the family and promote self-help for as long as the patient can manage. Simple occupation should be provided.

(3) Excitement and depression may be treated with tranquillisers and antidepressants as appropriate.

(4) In the later stages the patient will require full nursing care and attention.

Pick's disease

This condition was first described by Pick in 1892 and is similar to Alzheimer's disease in terms of age of onset, symptoms and prognosis.

1 The cause is unknown but genetic factors are important. The course is 2–10 years (the average is 7 years).

2 There is patchy degeneration of the cortex which affects both the grey and white matter. Neurological signs are minor or absent.

3 Moral and ethical values deteriorate easily. Dysphasia signs are minor or absent.

4 There is uninhibited behaviour totally out of character.

Management and treatment

The approach is the same as for Alzheimer's disease.

Senile dementia

This condition occurs in individuals at age 65 or over who show impairment in intellect, memory and personality due to brain damage and disease.

Differential diagnosis

Exclude other brain pathology (e.g. tumours and GPI), depression and neurotic conditions.

Signs and symptoms

1 Decline in intelligence with narrowing interests and difficulty in ability to solve problems.

2 Decline in memory, sometimes more for recent events than old ones.

3 Emotional disturbance with mood changes, irritability, agitation and depression.

4 Disturbed sleep rhythm.

5 Speech becomes muddled, vague and irrelevant.

6 Acute confusional states can occur with restlessness, wandering and disorientation.

7 Physical health deteriorates (e.g. weight reductions, increased risk of infections, incontinence) and personal hàbits decline (e.g. neglect of personal hygiene and appearance, messy eating habits).

Investigation—CAT scan

Since an important minority (10%) of patients have tumours or obstructive conditions CAT scan is a valuable, non-invasive method of investigation. It will also show cerebral atrophy and infarction.

Management and treatment

(1) Community care if possible (out-patient clinic and family service).

(2) If in hospital – supervision and observation.

(3) Maintain mobility (through remedial therapist, physiotherapy etc.).

(4) Drugs. (i) Sedatives for restlessness e.g. promazine (Sparine); (ii) nitrazepam or Chloral Hydrate at night.

(5) Correct vitamin deficiencies if necessary.

(6) Treat incontinence.

(7) Maintain physical health and prevent accidents.

(8) Occupation and recreation.

(9) Rehabilitation.

(10) Early discharge and social follow-up.

Nursing care is discussed at the end of this chapter.

Arteriosclerotic dementia

This dementia is associated with arteriosclerosis of the cerebral vessels and may be associated with hypertension. As a result of the arteriosclerotic pathology, the brain blood supply is reduced and damage may occur to the cortex and basal ganglia. Evidence of arteriosclerosis may be present in other parts of the body (e.g. enlargement of the heart, hypertension, coronary thrombosis).

Signs and Symptoms

1 These are similar to other dementias with memory deterioration, confusion, intellectual decline and so on.
2 It differs clinically from senile dementia in that:
    (a) Arteriosclerosis is always present.
    (b) It affects males more commonly.
    (c) It begins at an earlier age than senile dementia.
    (d) It is episodic rather than continuous.
    (e) It does not affect the personality until the disease is well advanced.
    (f) There may be other symptoms resulting from associated causes (e.g. headaches and dizziness from hypertension).

Management and treatment

(1) Hospitalisation.
(2) Drug therapy for hypertension (autonomic blocking agents).
(3) Rehabilitation – during phases of improvement the patient should be cared for at home. It is usually necessary to reduce work and responsibilities. In the later stages, when physical and mental deterioration worsen, full-time nursing care and attention are usually necessary.

Parkinsonism

The term 'Parkinsonism' comes from Parkinson's disease, (*paralysis agitans*), which is a degenerative disease of the basal ganglia. The cause is unknown and the disease occurs between the ages of 50–60 years.

Clinical features

(1) Muscular rigidity and shuffling gait. Pill rolling movement of fingers and tremor on movement and sleeping.
(2) Slow, slurred monotonous speech, and mask-like facial expression.
(3) Excessive salivation and sweating.
(4) Mental changes: resentment, depression, paranoid ideas and dementia.

Causes

(a) Encephalitis and cerebral arteriosclerosis.
(b) Haemorrhage into basal ganglia. Carbon monoxide and manganese poisoning.
(c) Induced by drugs such as trifluoperazine, thioridazine, fluphenazine (Moditen) and haloperidol (Serenace).

Prognosis

Parkinson's disease tends to be progressive until death but drug-induced symptoms can be relieved.

Management and treatment

(1) Keep patient active in the community for as long as possible.
(2) Prevent accidents due to patient's unsteadiness.
(3) Simple psychotherapy, physiotherapy and remedial therapy.
(4) Drug therapy.
  (a) Antidepressants if depression is a problem.
  (b) Anti-Parkinsonism drugs. (i) benzhezol (Artane), 2 − 5 mg three times daily; (ii) orphenadrine (Disipal), 50 mg three times daily; (iii) benztropine (Cogentin), 1 − 3 mg daily.
  (c) Nitrazepam for sleep.
(5) Occupational and recreational therapy.
Nursing care is discussed later in this chapter.

Note on extra-pyramidal reactions and phenothiazines

Psychotic patients on high doses of certain phenothiazines may exhibit extra-pyramidal reactions. Occasionally such reactions may exacerbate schizophrenic symptoms but if they are recognised and treated, the need for admission to hospital may be obviated. An outline of the more serious reactions includes:

Dyskinesia (dystonic reactions)

These are characterised by an abrupt onset of retrocollis, torticollis, facial grimacing and distortions, dysarthria, laboured breathing and involuntary muscle movements. Rarely, the patient may have an oculogyric crisis. Such an attack begins with a fixed stare for a few moments; the eyes are then rotated upwards, then to the side, and remain fixed in that position. At the same time the head is tilted backwards and laterally, the mouth open wide and the tongue protruding.

Akathisia

Akathisia or motor restlessness is often described as 'the jitters'. The patient feels compelled to pace the floor, shift his legs or tap his feet when sitting.

Parkinsonian side effects

Patients with Parkinsonism may exhibit rigidity of limbs, the cogwheel phenomenon, tremors, facial rigidity, poverty of movement, disturbance of gait and posture and drooling.

Treatment

Dystonic reactions can be relieved promptly by parenteral Benztropine Mesylate (Cogentin) or procyclidine (Kemadrin), the drugs taking effect within 10 minutes. Oral anti-Parkonsonism drugs such as Benztropine Mesylate (Cogentin), 1–3 mg daily, benzhexol (Artane), 6–15 mg daily, orphenadrine (Disipal), 200–300 mg daily or procyclidine (Kemadrin), 5 mg three times daily, usually prove effective in controlling day-to-day extrapyramidal symptoms.

Multiple sclerosis (disseminated sclerosis)

This is a progressive relapsing disease of unknown origin. Degeneration attacks the nerve fibres in different parts of the central nervous system. The condition is recurrent, with periods of remission decreasing as the degeneration advances. It occurs commonly in early and middle adulthood (between the ages 20–40). It is more common in females.

Signs and symptoms

Early stage
1 Visual disturbance, e.g. blurring vision and double vision.
2 Weakness in limbs, numbness and paraesthesiae.
3 Emotional changes – either euphoric or depressive.

Later stage

1 Ataxia (i.e. difficulty in co-ordinating).
2 Increased muscular tension, pain and incontinence.
3 Deterioration in intellectual functioning.
4 Finally, paraplegia and immobility.

Differential diagnosis

The vague physical symptoms with lack of neurological support (in the early stages) may indicate hysteria. Other organic brain diseases must be excluded also.

Management

(1) Community care and family support until the later stages.
(2) In some cases, rest in hospital during acute attacks.
(3) Drug therapy. (i) Corticotrophin (ACTH) injections may help during acute attacks. (ii) Anti-spasmodic drugs for spasticity (e.g. diazepam).
(4) Physiotherapy and remedial therapy for stiffness, and walking aids if necessary.
(5) Occupational and recreational therapy.
(6) Counselling, reassurance and support for patient's family.
(7) Prevention of limb deformity during early attacks and full nursing care and attention during terminal stages.

General paralysis of the insane

Ten to fifteen years after the initial infection, the syphilis spirochaete (*Treponema pallidum*) may attack the meninges and brain substance. Brain changes may include thickening of the meninges, atrophy of the convolutions and dilation of the ventricles.

Clinical features

Both physical and mental symptoms are present but the main feature is the progressive destruction of mental functions.

Mental

(1) Evidence of memory disturbance for recent events.
(2) Euphoria, delusions of grandeur and general manic type behaviour.

(3) Apathy, dullness and intellectual deterioration.
(4) Irritability and sudden aggression or bizarre behaviour.
(5) Lack of concentration and further decline in memory.

Physical
(1) Argyll-Robertson pupils, i.e. small unequal pupils which do not react to light but do react to accommodation.
(2) Coarse tremor of face, lips and tongue.
(3) Muscular weakness of limbs, (spasticity) and incontinence.
(4) Ataxia and tremor of the hands.
(5) Epileptic fits may occur.
(6) Paralysis may occur (hemiplegia).
(7) More progressive and marked dementia with paralysis and blindness.

Differential diagnosis

The condition may resemble other psychiatric conditions such as hypomania, confusion, schizophrenia, depression, pre-senile dementia, cerebral arteriosclerosis and alcoholic states.

Diagnosis

(1) Blood tests Wassermann reaction (WR) and Kahn.
(2) Cerebrospinal fluid examination using Wassermann reaction and sometimes Lange's Colloidal Gold Curve Test.

Management and treatment

(1) Rest, investigation and observation.
(2) Procaine penicillin 1.2 g daily by i.m. injection for 10 days.
(3) Post penicillin follow-up (regular checks at periodic intervals to ensure treatment effectiveness). This may be necessary for several years afterwards.
(4) Prevention of physical deterioration and promotion of self-help.
(5) Occupation and recreation.
The prognosis is hopeful if the condition is diagnosed early and prompt treatment is given. Patients who are in an advanced stage of deterioration will require full nursing care and attention. Tranquillisers may be necessary for advanced symptoms.

Tabes Dorsalis

This chronic syphilitic disease damages the sensory nerve roots of the dorsal columns of the spinal cord. It occurs between 14 and 24 years after the initial infection and affects about 4 per cent of syphilitic sufferers. Once established, the disease is showly progressive and crippling over several years.

Signs and symptoms

1 Pain in the legs (rheumatic type) and lightning pains are the first symptoms. The patient experiences fleeting stabbing pains lasting from seconds to days.
2 Heavy numb feeling in the limbs.
3 Impotence and incontinence.
4 Ataxia and eventually inability to walk without the aid of sticks.
5 Rombergism — an inability to stand without swaying with the eyes closed and the feet placed together.
6 Double vision and blindness in some cases.
7 Charcot joints — painless enlargement of the joints (usually the ankle, knee, hip and upper limb joints).

Diagnosis

(1) Characteristic signs and symptoms to be checked.
(2) WR and Kahn blood tests and CSF examination may be made.

Management and treatment

(1) Rest in hospital.
(2) Drug therapy. (i) Daily injections of procaine penicillin (1.2 g daily) for a period of 10–14 days. A second course may be necessary three months later. (ii) Analgesics (Codeine) for tabetic pains.
(3) Regular follow-ups to check that infection is arrested.

Note on organic brain disorders

In addition to the conditions discussed in this chapter, there are numerous other conditions which affect the nervous system (either directly or indirectly) and cause psychiatric symptoms. These include:

(1) Cerebral tumours and abscesses.

(2) Brain injuries (e.g. post traumatic dementia and punch drunkenness).

(3) Pellagra and cerebral anoxia.

(4) Hypothyroidism (myxoedema) and thyrotoxicosis (see Chapter 28).

(5) Hypoglycaemia and uraemia.

(6) Chemical poisoning (e.g. lead, mercury and phosphorus).

(7) Vitamin B_{12} deficiency.

(8) Meningitis and encephalitis.

For information on these specific conditions the student should refer to a textbook on psychiatry (see Recommended Reading List).

Nursing care of organic conditions

It is a misconception to view the patient with dementia as being a hopeless chronic case. While it is true that some may never recover completely, many have sufficient brain function remaining to enable them to learn self-help again. Even those with progressive dementia must be encouraged to use their remaining abilities for as long as is possible. The nurse should look on the bright side in her relationship with the patient. She should be positive in her attitude and treat each patient as an individual regardless of his personality deterioration and prognosis.

There are many aspects of care which may include the following:

Reducing invalidism. The nursing effort should commence with the patient's admission to hospital. The patient should be encouraged to develop his remaining abilities and the nurse should avoid doing things for him which he is capable of doing for himself. Initially he will require support and reassurance but this should be combined with suggestions that he should maintain correct habits regarding personal hygiene, appearance, eating etiquette and regular elimination. Participation in therapeutic activities is essential to combat personality malfunction.

Disabling aspects of the patient's condition require prompt attention. Remedial therapy, speech therapy, and physiotherapy are resources which can facilitate the patient's capacity to function. Disorientation should not be allowed to consolidate, and persistent explanation and repetition will do much to reorientate the individual to persons, time and events. The nurse will require patience to remotivate the patient to self-help so that invalidism and dependence are reduced.

Physical care. The patient's neglect of physical health may lead to rapid deterioration and further disablement. The nurse must guard against this by ensuring attention to basic physical needs as outlined in Chapter 7. Careful observation should be made to detect early coughs which may lead to serious respiratory tract infections. The more serious cases of dementia may require more detailed physical attention. In the terminal stage of illness, many become bedridden and need assistance with their personal hygiene, feeding and bathing. Regular attention to pressure areas is important and every effort should be made to prevent sores.

Helping the relatives. It is not easy for relatives to accept the outcome of dementias which are progressive and may end with premature death. Initially they will receive explanation and support from the doctor in charge of the patient's case. Thereafter, the nursing staff must do all they can to aid the relatives. They should be encouraged to involve themselves in the patient's care and many feel happier in doing so. Some like to help by taking home the patient's personal laundry and others may spend their free time visiting or taking the patient for walks or drives in the country.

Relatives dependent on the 'breadwinner' should be introduced to the social worker so that supportive services can be explained to them. In cases where the patient is well enough to be at home, arrangements should be made to help the family to cope. Many services, such as community psychiatric nurses, district nurses, home helps and the provision of Meals on Wheels, disposable laundry, wheelchairs, walking aids etc., exist to help relatives who wish to care for the patient at home. The relatives should be reassured that they may return the patient to hospital if they wish to go away on holiday or if the patient becomes too difficult to manage.

24

Confusion and Physical Handicaps

Confusion

The confused patient cannot grasp what he sees; he is mixed up and muddled; he is perplexed; he may be unaware of his surrounding; he is not sure of his identity, whereabouts or the time; he keeps forgetting things; he is indecisive and cannot pay attention to anything. In extreme cases he may be hallucinated. On the whole, it is a very unreal, insecure and frightening world for the patient.

Acute confusional state

Acute confusion may have a rapid onset and may also be referred to as delirium, symptomatic psychosis, or toxic-exhaustive psychosis. The condition is characterised by disorientation in person, time and place, restlessness, frightening visual hallucinations, illusions, neglect of physical health and appearance, and deteriorated personal habits.

Causes

(a) Infections which produce toxins and exhaustion e.g. pneumonia, influenza, typhoid fever, septicaemia, uremia.
(b) Head injury – on regaining consciousness the patient may be very confused.
(c) Chemical – drug or alcohol intoxication and following withdrawal of such substances.
(d) Cerebral tumours and cerebrovascular accident (stroke).
(e) Metabolic and endocrine dysfunction e.g. diabetic hypoglycaemia.
(f) Post-operative exhaustion or other complications.
(g) Puerperal psychosis, epilepsy and dementias.

Long-term confusion

Patients with senility and progressive dementias may be confused for longer periods. In the later stages of progressive organic brain diseases, confusion may be a permanent symptom with only very occasional lucid intervals.

Management and treatment of confusional states

(1) Rest, observation and prevention from injury. Attention to physical care. Repeated explanation and reassurance. The patient should be observed and prevented from injury. Attention should be paid to physical care and he should be made to rest. Repeated explanation and reassurance should be given.

(2) Acute confusion is usually reversible. Treatment is specific and related to the underlying cause, e.g. infections will require antibiotics or epilepsy will be treated with anticonvulsants.

(3) Sedation, in acute states, with noisiness and restlessness.
(i) Chlorpromazine (Largactil) 100 mg three times daily;
(ii) night sedation – nitrazepam (Mogadon) to promote sleep.

Nursing care of the confused patient

Environment. The patient should be nursed in a small ward with a fairly simple layout. Ward directions and facilities should be well signposted, as this makes it easier for the patient to find his way about and to understand his surroundings. Good lighting is important and shadows should be minimised as they will worsen the patient's confusion. Floors should be non-slip and steps may cause the patient to stumble. Confused patients may interfere with fires, switches etc., therefore, fire guards should be locked.

Nursing relationship. The nurse should adopt a quiet, friendly approach to the patient; she must be tolerant and explain things over and over until the patient grasps their meaning; she should stay with the patient until he settles on the ward. A friendly familiar face gives the patient something to hold on to; therefore, the relatives are encouraged to visit frequently and there should be no restrictions on time.

The nurse should practise a slow rigid regime for the confused patient, this will help him to grasp routines. The patient should not be rushed, plenty of time is needed for eating, dressing and so on. Changes should be avoided as they will further muddle him. Allow the patient to sit at the same place every day for his meals, sleep in the same part of the ward, and so on. Slowly he will begin to grasp things and feel less confused; he will gradually learn to recognise the nurse's face, the table he sits at for lunch, the bed he sleeps in, and so on.

Observation and supervision are important. The nurse must observe for any signs of physical deterioration and attend to

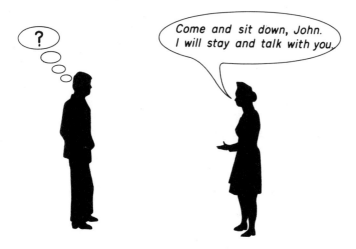

Fig. 24.1 The confused patient may be frightened

physical needs. The patient will require supervision because of the risk of injuries and wandering. Care needs to be taken with the patient's smoking habits as they present a risk of fire or self-injury. The nurse should help the patient during bathtime to prevent scalding or other injury.

As the patient learns to understand and recover, the nurse can further develop the relationship to encourage participation in rehabilitation. The whole approach to nursing the confused patient should be a step-by-step process. With each step to recovery, the nurse should be working towards her next objective. A slow tempo should prevail and, at all times, the nurse must be conscious of factors in the patient's illness and the ward environment which may increase confusion.

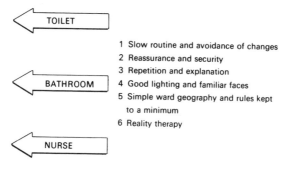

Fig. 24.2 Reducing confusion

Physical handicaps and mental disorder

The nurse may encounter a variety of physical handicaps among patients in psychiatric hospitals. These may include: paralysis, loss of limb, deafness, blindness and speech defects.

Paralysis

Patients may have paralysis of one or more limbs due to factors such as injuries, hysteria, strokes, LSD mishaps and so on. It is important for the nurse to consider that the paralysis may not be permanent, and therefore, she must ensure that the limb does not become deformed. The limb should be maintained in the correct position and physiotherapy applied daily. The patient should be prevented from becoming a 'psychological cripple' with encouragement and confidence to adjust to life. He should participate in social and recreational activities and his rehabilitation must include learning or retraining in an occupation suitable for his functioning and disability.

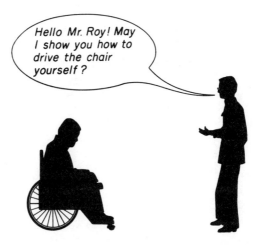

Fig. 24.3   Preventing psychological invalidism

Loss of limb

Patients who lose limbs require a great deal of reassurance and support. The nurse must help them by instilling confidence in their ability to overcome the disability. The inherent danger is that such patients may feel sorry for themselves and expect the nursing staff to do everything for them. Dependence must be discouraged and the patient must be encouraged to face the future in a positive way. The patient's rehabilitation should include introduction to groups and organisations which specialise in helping people with such problems. The patient will be fitted with an artificial limb and encouraged to use it.

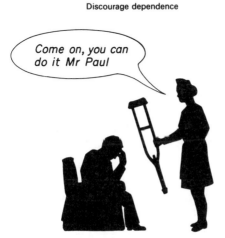

Discourage dependence

The danger is that such patients may feel sorry for themselves and develop dependence on the nurse

Fig. 24.4 Loss of limb

Deafness

Partial deafness can be helped with the use of a hearing aid. Some patients with hearing difficulties may become paranoid and the nurse should be aware of factors in the environment which may contribute to the patient's suspicion. Those with severe deafness should be taught to lip-read and the nurse should facilitate this when articulating to the patient. The nurse should introduce the patient to television news bulletins which are read especially for deaf people. Also, there are various voluntary groups and associations which exist to help people with deafness. The nurse should be familiar with the local agent and invite him along to meet the patient.

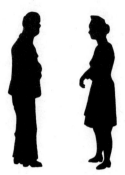

The nurse should face the patient and speak clearly
to facilitate lip reading

Fig. 24.5   Lip reading

Blindness

The darkness of being blind is difficult for some patients to come to terms with. The nurse must give them confidence to face life with this disability. The patient will need to learn braille and should be provided with a braille library. The nurse must be prepared (with the patient's permission) to read non-braille correspondence to him when necessary. There are many braille games on the market and these should be available for the patient's use. Part of the patient's rehabilitation should include introduction to a guide dog association before he leaves the hospital.

Speech defects

Many speech defects can be helped by speech therapy. Patients who are unable to communicate verbally should be taught sign

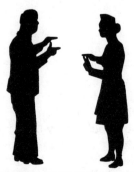

The enthusiastic nurse will learn simple sign language
to understand the patient's communication

Fig. 24.6   Sign language

language. Also, the nurse should ensure that the patient is provided with a pencil, notepaper and a bell to facilitate communication. In some cases the enthusiastic nurse will learn simple sign language to interpret the patient's communication.

25
Epilepsy

Epilepsy is a disease in which abnormal electrical discharge in the brain results in disturbance of movement, feeling and consciousness. Between four and six people in every thousand have epileptic fits at some time in their lives. The abnormal electrical waves can be seen in the electroencephalogram (EEG).

Recognising types of epilepsy

There are several kinds of fit. Some patients may have the same fit all their lives while others may have several kinds.

The grand mal fit

This passes through a series of stages:

(1) *Aura.* The fit may be preceded by an aura which may consist of flashing lights, forced movements, or vague sensations and emotions.

(2) *Tonic stage.* The fit proper begins with generalised contraction of all voluntary muscles and loss of consciousness. As a result the patient falls to the ground and lies rigid. Respiration stops and the patient may make a shrieking noise as air is expelled from the lungs. This stage of rigidity and absent breathing lasts about 30 seconds.

(3) *Clonic stage.* This succeeds the tonic phase and may last from one to five minutes. In this stage the patient remains unconscious but breathing commences again. The muscles contract and relax causing the limbs to thrash about and the trunk to jerk up and down. This stage may alarm someone who has not seen a fit before. Frothing at the mouth and incontinence may occur.

(4) *Post-convulsive stage.* Following the clonic phase the patient appears exhausted, may sleep, and before regaining full consciousness may be confused and wander about. In some cases a post epileptic automatism may follow a fit; the patient may perform acts such as undressing or he may become disturbed and violent. During automatism the patient is not aware of what he is doing.

Petit mal (minor) fit

In this attack the patient has only a momentary loss of consciousness. He does not fall down, convulse or wet himself. He simply breaks conversation or stops what he is doing for a second or two, then resumes where he left off. The whole episode is over in seconds.

Jacksonian epilepsy

The fit begins locally as a muscular contraction in a part of the body – the thumb, the big toes, or a corner of the mouth. It can be stopped by squeezing the contracting part, but in some instances it can develop into a grand mal fit.

Temporal lobe epilepsy

This is produced by lesions in the temporal lobe and shows as impairment of consciousness, disorientation, dream states and memory disturbances.

Status epilepticus

This is repeated grand mal attacks in rapid succession. The patient remains unconscious and continues to fit for periods varying from an hour to several weeks.

Causes

(a) Heredity factors.
(b) Brain damage resulting from anoxia and injuries.
(c) Physical diseases. In young children convulsions occur during fevers. Convulsion may be secondary to factors such as fatigue, over-hydration, hypoglycaemia and uraemia.
(d) Epileptic convulsions are common in some mental handicap states e.g. epiloia.
(e) Unknown cause – idiopathic epilepsy.

Fit patterns

Some patients may have their fits in groups, e.g., an individual may have four convulsions one day and one the next. He may then have no more for several weeks until he has another attack of convulsions in two or three days. Some patients may always have their fit during the night and never in day-time while others may have them regularly before evening supper.

Complications of major convulsions

1 *Injuries.* These may depend on where the patient is when he fits. For example, it is not unusual to observe scar injuries on chronic epileptics. Injuries may be more severe if the patient falls near a fire and sustains a burn or if he is working at a height and falls to the ground.

2 *Tongue-biting* is a common complication in the major convulsion.

3 *Fractures and dislocations.* Fractures are rare but dislocation of the shoulder and jaw occur more easily.

4 *Suffocation.* The patient may choke during the convulsion if he has food in his mouth when the fit commences. During the night the patient may suffocate on a soft pillow; therefore, it is important to use hard pillows on the patient's bed.

Differential diagnosis

1. Distinguish from hysteria (see Chapter 14).

2. Syncopal (fainting) attacks may occur in heart disease and anxiety states.

3. Narcolepsy. This is an invincible desire to sleep for short intervals which may overcome the patient several times a day and cause him to fall down. This condition may be associated with acute depression and is treated with Dexamphetamine Sulphate, 5 mg twice daily up to 60 mg daily.

Psychiatric aspects of epilepsy

(1) Confusional attacks – a period of acute confusion may follow a major attack and automatisms may occur.

(2) Paranoid psychosis. Long-standing epileptics may develop a psychotic disorder which usually takes the form of a chronic paranoid state featuring delusions of persecution, ideas of reference and hallucinations.

(3) Aggressive outbursts may follow major convulsions.

(4) Intellectual deterioration may occur after many years of major attacks.

(5) Depression and neurotic reactions because of this disability are not uncommon.

Management and treatment for epilepsy

(1) Anti-convulsants can be administered: (i) phenytoin sodium (Epanutin), (ii) carbamazepine (Tegretol), (iii) phenobarbitone

(Luminal), (iv) primidone (Mysoline) for grand mal epilepsy; (v) ethosuximide (Zarontin) for petit mal epilepsy; (vi) sulthiame (Ospolot), (vii) sodium valproate (Epilim) for all forms of epilepsy; (viii) benzodiazepines such as clonazepam (Rivotril) and diazepam (Valium) are also used to control severe convulsions (status epilepticus).

(2) Tranquillisers for psychiatric complications: (i) diazepam (Valium); (ii) chlorpromazine (Largactil).

(3) Surgery. Surgical removal of the part of the brain responsible for focal epilepsy may be used (providing the removal of the affected area can be done without crippling the patient).

Management and treatment of status epilepticus

The onset of status epilepticus calls for emergency treatment:

(1) Ensure a clear airway.

(2) Intravenous injections of diazepam (Valium) given slowly with close monitoring of ventilatory function.

(3) Observations of TPR, drug administration, fluid input and output, and occurrence of fits. These should all be carefully recorded. Elevation of temperature may indicate pneumonia and this may call for prompt antibiotic therapy.

(4) Full nursing care and attention to diet.

The electroencephalogram (EEG): It is an essential test for epilepsy in all ages and is usually performed after at least four hours fasting as EEG abnormalities show up more clearly with a low blood sugar. The EEG may accurately pin-point the part of the cerebral cortex producing the epilepsy and in some cases it may reveal whether the epilepsy is symptomatic of brain disease (e.g. cerebral tumour).

General discussion on epilepsy

Epilepsy is still a social stigma as well as a disability. Epileptics may not be allowed to drive vehicles or hold a job where fits are likely to have a dangerous consequence. Some employers are reluctant to employ epileptics and in the public mind, epilepsy is still mistakenly connected with crime, degeneration and low intelligence. It is not surprising, therefore, that epileptics may react to their illness by becoming anxious, sullen and embittered.

Psychiatric problems may result from epilepsy. Patients may be depressed and irritable for several days prior to fits. In middle-aged patients with temporal lobe epilepsy, paranoid psychosis sometimes develops. Epileptic personality formation may be seen in terms of stated claims that such patients are egocentric, hypochondriacal, moody, unpleasant, touchy and liable to outbursts of temper.

Nursing care

The majority of people with epilepsy are in the community. Only a small minority with frequent fits or personality disturbances are hospitalised.

A detailed nursing assessment should be conducted to identify the patient's needs and risk factors as described in Chapter 11. Particular consideration is given to the implications of the condition for the patient's activities of daily living. Important points which frequently require consideration when planning nursing care include:

1 Coping with major attacks. When a patient has a grand mal attack the nurse should try to break his fall. He should be allowed to lie where he has fallen (except where it would be dangerous not to move him) and a cushion should be placed under his head. Tight clothing should be loosened about the patient's neck and waist. His body movements should not be restrained but he should be kept under observation until the seizure is completed. The patient should be offered a bath on recovery and any injuries resulting from his fall should be observed and treated. A full report of the incident should be made to the charge nurse.

2 Report on observations. The nurse should note behaviour or incidents prior to the attack, duration of unconsciousness, type of seizure, time and place of occurrence, past behaviour and whether there was incontinence or injury.

3 Considered nursing approach. The environment should not be seen to discriminate against the epileptic by imposing restrictions which reflect the nurse's over-concern for the patient's safety. This approach to management may continually make the patient feel an outsider in the eyes of the staff and other patients. He should be managed just like any other patient who is also an individual with specific needs which are related to his illness. There is nothing outstanding concerning patient activities in a modern mental hospital which should exclude the epileptic on the grounds that it is not safe. To exclude the epileptic merely helps to reinforce his sensitivity. He can, e.g., participate in work therapy, recreational activities, group activities, patient outings and so on. Quite rightly one can add that he should not work with dangerous machines, climb ladders, bath alone, sleep on soft pillows and so on.

4 Prevention of fits. Nursing care should involve an awareness of factors which may help to reduce the incidence of fits. It is generally believed that sudden changes in ward environment, stress, friction in relationships, irregular medication and constipation may bring on attacks. The nurse must reduce or eliminate these factors and if the patient's fits are to remain controlled when he is discharged, the patient should be helped to understand their significance.

Drugs are the most widely used method of preventing and controlling attacks. The nurse must be observant for side effects and the patient will require education in their administration and safety before being discharged.

5 Rehabilitation. A good varied programme of therapeutic activities is important in the general care and rehabilitation of the epileptic patient. This is necessary for the patient's self-esteem, social acceptance, and return to society. It is also an important factor in reducing frictions, preventing boredom, and easing the frustrations of his circumstances. The selected activities should follow the same guidelines which have been outlined for the care of other patients in previous chapters. During rehabilitation the patient may be introduced to an epileptic association if he so wishes.

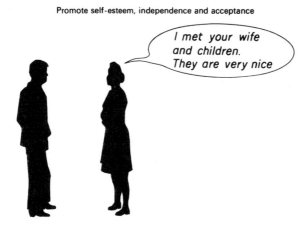

Promote self-esteem, independence and acceptance

discourage self-pity, bitterness and a 'chip on the shoulder'

Fig. 25.1 Rehabilitation

26
Mental Handicaps

'Mentally handicapped' is the term most generally used to describe people whose learning abilities, maturation and social functioning are retarded to varying degrees. Some of them may also have physical defects. There is a tendency to classify them only according to their intellectual level, which is below what is considered to be normal. Some mentally handicapped people are not badly affected; they are educable and will manage to hold down a job of work and achieve marriage. Others, however, will never be able to do this, requiring intensive training even to master basic communication and personal functioning (see pages 181–2). (For legal definitions, refer to Mental Health Acts in Chapter 32, page 228.)

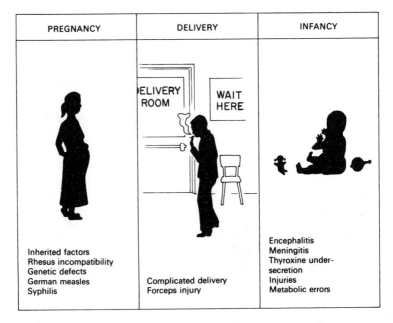

PREGNANCY	DELIVERY	INFANCY
Inherited factors Rhesus incompatibility Genetic defects German measles Syphilis	Complicated delivery Forceps injury	Encephalitis Meningitis Thyroxine under- secretion Injuries Metabolic errors

Fig. 26.1 Causes of mental handicap

Recognising mental handicap

Paediatricians, health visitors, midwives or the infant's mother may be the first to recognise that a child is mentally handicapped.

Specific physical features may be recognisable at birth but others such as slowness to walk and speak may only show later in the child's development. Physical and mental assessment will confirm diagnosis. In some borderline cases the condition may remain unnoticed until adulthood when a court appearance or some other deviation may indicate a mental handicap.

There are many types of mental handicap and they include conditions such as Down's syndrome, cretinism, microcephaly and phenylketonuria.

Classification of mental handicaps

People with mental handicaps have retarded intellectual functioning which becomes apparent during early life. Because of this, classification is most frequently correlated with a person's intelligence quotient (IQ), see pp. 186, 282. It is well known, however, that these tests in people with mental handicap can be unreliable and that other features of their personalities and abilities must be taken into account when assessing their potential for development. Classifications vary between countries but categories can be roughly defined as:

1 People with an IQ of between 50 and 70. They may appear normal in infancy but will be slow to walk, talk and fend for themselves. They do poorly at school and may leave early to settle in a routine job which calls for little intelligence. Many of these people with 'mental handicap' marry but usually to someone with a similar intelligence level.

Some of them may have unstable personalities and this creates more problems for the individual and his family. They may require special education in a junior training centre or Special Care School. On leaving school they may have difficulty holding a job. A minority may break the law occasionally and end up in youth custody or prison. Many have difficulties in following complicated instructions (e.g. form-filling, tax demands, pay slips and so on).

2 People with an IQ ranging from 0–50. They are usually said to have severe mental handicap. People with such low intelligence may also have physical deformities. They are likely to be mishapen in physique and features. Their eyes may be slanting (as in Down's syndrome) and some may be deaf or blind and have speech difficulties.

Mentally handicapped people within this IQ range are more dependent on others for their social, personal and educational functions. Some can be taught to wash and feed themselves but will become careless if supervision is lacking. Teaching and training for them has to be slow and simple. Many can be taught to speak short simple sentences and recognise their name, coins and words. They tend to excel at repetitive tasks.

Severely handicapped people may be completely dependent on others. Many are incontinent and have to be fed, washed and dressed.

3 Under the provisions of the Mental Health Act 1983, a small number of mentally handicapped people with additional behaviour disorders can be subject to compulsory admission into safe-keeping or guardianship. This is dealt with in Chapter 32.

Some conditions causing mental handicap are described below:

Down's syndrome

Incidence

One baby in every 600 is born with Down's syndrome.

Cause

People with Down's syndrome have 47 chromosomes in their cells instead of the normal 46. It is believed that the extra chromosome causes the condition. Pre-disposing factors are increased maternal age and a family history of the syndrome.

Clinical features

(1) 'Mongolian' features with slanting eyes and a round flat face.
(2) Stunted growth, short neck and trunk. Misshapen ears and large tongue.
(3) Small round head with no occipital protuberance and coarse skin with sparse hair. Obesity in adulthood.
(4) Poor sexual development and poor circulation (peripheral cyanosis).
(5) Single crease across palm (instead of two) and deformity of the little finger.

IQ range

Ranges from 25–50 but a few may have above 50.

Complications

People with Down's syndrome often suffer from congenital heart disease and epilepsy, and are susceptible to pneumonia and leukaemia. Half die before school age and few live to old age.

Phenylketonuria

This is an inherited metabolic disorder due to a failure of the liver to convert phenylalanine (an amino acid found in all natural protein foods) into tryosine. The phenylalanine accumulates in the blood and damages the brain. The substance is eventually excreted in the urine.

Diagnosis

Phenistix urine test and the Guthrie blood test should be made.

Clinical features

(1) Normal at birth but signs of slow development become apparent in infancy.
(2) Generally blue eyes and fair hair.
(3) Patchy eczema.
(4) Epileptic fits may occur.
(5) Over-active and twitching mannerisms.

Incidence

One in 20 000 persons is affected.

Treatment

Treatment is directed at reducing the level of phenylalanine in the blood by giving a phenylalanine low diet and preparations which contain the enzyme which will metabolise phenylalanine.

Cretinism

Cause

Cretinism results from an under-secretion of thyroid hormone in children.

Clinical features

(1) Recognised in early months of life. The baby is lethargic, cries little and is a poor feeder.
(2) Thick dry skin, brittle hair.
(3) Sub-normal temperature and pulse.
(4) Stunted growth (cretin dwarf).

Treatment

Early recognition is important and prompt administration of thyroxine, 0.025 mg daily. If mental development is retarded, it will always be so, and there is no 'cure'.

Kernicterus

Cause

This is caused by Rhesus incompatibility. This is produced when a Rhesus (Rh) negative woman is impregnated by a Rhesus (Rh) positive man. The baby inherits the father's (Rh positive) blood and the mother's blood damages the infant's; thus the developing brain may be deprived of oxygen and nutrients.

Clinical features

(1) Severe jaundice in the newborn baby. Some may die prematurely.
(2) Twitching, fits and vomiting.
(3) Retardation, epilepsy and deafness.

Treatment (preventive)

(1) Rh negative mothers should have regular blood checks for positive antibodies during the later stages of pregnancy.
(2) Induced delivery if necessary.
(3) Intra-uterine exchange transfusions of Rh negative blood.

Management and treatment of mentally handicapped patients

(1) Emphasis on community care and special education.
(2) Hospitalisation if the case is too severe to be managed in the community. A rehabilitative approach is needed.

(3) Drugs – as required for aggression or epilepsy e.g. anti-convulsants and tranquillisers.

(4) Speech therapy, physiotherapy, occupation and recreation.

(5) Counselling and reassurance for patient's family.

(6) Diet or hormones (e.g. phenylketonuria and cretinism).

(7) Behaviour modification is used with success for improving deteriorated habits, aggression and so on. This is based on reward systems for good behaviour and disapproval or withholding rewards for bad behaviour.

(8) Habit training may be useful for the more deteriorated patients as they tend to do well at repetitive actions.

(9) Social skills training.

Social care of the mentally handicapped

There should be a community emphasis on caring for the mentally handicapped, because such children will develop best in the company of their own family. Initially the parents will require a great deal of explanation and support in coming to terms with their child's handicap and later a great deal of concern and anxiety may result from the child's social inefficiency and lack of independence.

Health visitors, community nurses, social workers, parent associations and health clinics, all have an important role to play in assisting the family to bring up their child, but this should be seen as supportive aid rather than professional interference.

From the age of 5 until 16, the Education Authority is responsible for education and training. Special schools are available which specialise in helping the handicapped child. These schools adapt to the child's needs and expertly trained teachers give them more attention than is possible in the ordinary school system. Children who live a distance from the school receive assisted transport from the Education Authority.

On leaving school at 16 years, the young person will be helped to find employment suitable to his abilities. For those who are unable to hold down a job, more training will be provided by adult centres and sheltered employment units. The latter agencies will continue occupational and social competence training, thus enabling the young person to gain further experience and confidence to face the future as a citizen.

Hospital care of the mentally handicapped

Severely handicapped persons may be admitted to hospital because they cannot be cared for, or receive the training they require, in the community. The aims of the hospital should be to prepare them for a return to outside life as soon as possible. In the pursuit of these aims, the nurse is a key factor. Her attitude to nursing and rehabilitation should be a positive one; she should be objective and take care not to allow over-protective attitudes to influence her role; she should be skilled in the arts of basic teaching and be open to influences which will help her patients to learn; she should have a good knowledge of the hospital personnel and departments so that she can relate them to her nursing programme and local community facilities.

IQ range of the mentally handicapped

A wide range of IQs may be recorded in people who are regarded as mentally handicapped. There is no sharp dividing line in terms of IQ between normal intelligence and mental handicap, but clinical practice sets the upper limits of mental handicaps at about IQ 70–80. In practice people with IQs between 0–50 fall within the definition of severe mental handicap. There is no sharp dividing line as such between severe mental handicap and mental handicap.

27

Psychiatric Disorders of Childbirth, Childhood and Adolescence

Childbirth

Mental illness during pregnancy is no more a risk than at other times but following childbirth, attacks of neurosis or psychosis are not uncommon.

Neuroses are not common but when they occur they are usually confined to persons who have had a previous neurotic breakdown or have an existing neurotic predisposition. The stress of childbirth and the new responsibility of bringing up a child may be a stress factor in causing the breakdown. The patient will present the usual features of a neurotic patient and the symptoms may be of an anxiety state, obsessional state or hysterical reaction. Treatment will be on the same lines as previously discussed for neurosis but a great deal of reassurance and support will be necessary to allay any fears or anxieties about the child's health and welfare or the patient's abilities for motherhood. Training, advice and support from the health visitor and district midwives can be very reassuring and confidence-boosting.

Puerperal psychosis

Severe forms of this disorder occur in about 1 – 800 live births and may begin in an acute way in the first 7– 10 days of the puerperium (which is the period of confinement following childbirth and regarded by obstetricians as lasting 10 days). In some cases, however, the onset is later than the puerperium (breakdowns may occur between 6–12 weeks after delivery) but they are also described as puerperal.

Clinical features

Depression is the most common puerperal state but mixed schizo-effective reactions are also common.
(1) Onset is usually acute.
(2) Loss of feelings for baby and husband.

(3) Perplexity and disorientation in severe cases.
(4) Delusions and hallucinations.
(5) Suicidal tendencies.
(6) Neglect of personal appearance and hygiene.
(7) Loss of appetite and sleep.
(8) Restlessness and confusion.
(9) Infanticidal tendencies. (Infanticide is the term used when a mother kills her child within 12 months of birth. It is differentiated from murder if it is committed whilst the mother is mentally unbalanced. D. J. West in his book 'Murder Followed by Suicide' shows that in a study of 45 child victims only 11 were under one year old.)

Management and treatment

In hospital
(1) The child may be admitted with the mother if the hospital has a nursery or mother and baby unit. Alternatively the child may be cared for by relatives or the husband may prefer to manage with support from midwifery, home help, and social worker services. In some cases it may be necessary to put the child into local authority care but whenever possible the mother/child link must be renewed.
(2) Psychotherapy.
(3) Drugs – antidepressants, tranquillisers and night sedation.
(4) Electroconvulsive therapy (ECT) in some cases.
(5) Mothering. The patient must be encouraged to take an interest in her baby and continue with mothering. Initially it may be necessary to do this under supervision and later when the patient leaves hospital she will need the support of health visitors, social workers and so on. Puerperal psychosis can have a traumatic effect on the husband so counselling and reassurance will be necessary.

Nursing care

The acute puerperal patient will require the nursing care detailed for other psychotic reactions outlined in previous chapters. This will include:
1 Immediate physical care and attention to diet, personal hygiene and appearance.
2 Observation and prevention of suicide and infanticide.

3 Reassurance and support.
4 Encouraging family interests and mothering.
5 Rehabilitation and preparation for discharge.

Note on abortion and sterilisation

Abortion may be advised on psychiatric grounds if the mental
health of the mother is likely to be worsened by the pregnancy
continuing. Abortion may also be recommended if the foetus is
thought to be abnormal or if it is likely that another child will
adversely affect the mother and other children within the family.

There may be psychiatric complications following abortions in
some patients. For example, Ekbald found in a study of 479
patients who had had abortions that 11 per cent had psychiatric
disturbance and 25 per cent regretted the abortion.

Sterilisation may also be advised if it is likely that further
pregnancies will endanger the mental health of the mother or other
children within the family.

Disorders of childhood

Most psychiatric conditions in children arise from difficulties
within the home or at school. The following disorders are
common in child psychiatry.

Nocturnal enuresis (bed-wetting)

Normally a child becomes dry at the age of 3 but a diagnosis of
bed-wetting should not be made until the child is 5 years old.

Causes

(a) Emotional threats or insecurity e.g. the arrival of a new baby
or parental separation.
(b) Low intelligence and lack of training by parents.
(c) Following operations or genito-urinary infection.
(d) Organic disease may be a cause in 5 per cent of cases.

Management and treatment

(1) Toilet training (potting) after a few hours in bed.
(2) Conditioned reflex therapy using bed pad and bell attach-

ment. The bell wakes the child when the pad is wetted and it is hoped that the regular nightly waking will build up a conditioned reflex against bed-wetting.

(3) Investigations on urine to exclude infection.

(4) Psychotherapy and family therapy to improve parent-child relationships in some cases.

Nail-biting and thumb-sucking

These may be normal in infancy but may persist in children who are unhappy or worried.

Temper tantrums and breath-holding

Temper tantrums may occur whereby the child screams, kicks, bangs his head or throws himself to the floor. The attack is followed by sobbing and in a few minutes all is well again.

Breath-holding is a state whereby the child holds his breath until he goes blue in the face and falls unconscious. In a few moments the child relaxes and breathing commences again. An attack can be alarming to observe and a child may have several attacks each day.

Stammering

Stammering may commence between the third and sixth years of life and again at puberty. In severe cases it may be prolonged and persist into adult life as a serious handicap. Treatment is by speech therapy and psychotherapy.

Tics

Tics are involuntary movements of groups of muscles. The movements are purposeless and may take the form of blinking, sniffing, shrugging, grunting, head jerking and so on. Excitement or attempts to suppress the tics may make them worse. If the child is left alone without fuss the tics nearly always disappear.

Psychosomatic disorders

Anxious children may have pains and headaches but some may develop illnesses such as asthma, eczema and ulcerative colitis.

Neurotic disorders

Neuroses may occur in children and they include anxiety states, obsessional states and hysteria. School phobia may occur in some children whereby, through fear of school, they play truant or refuse to leave for school.

Childhood psychosis

Psychosis is rare in childhood but occasionally depression or mania may occur. The conditions are usually milder than in adulthood but suicide may occur during acute depressions.

Autism

This is a condition which may develop about the age of 2 years. It is not unlike schizophrenia. The condition was first described by Kanner (1943) and consists of an inability to respond to the environment.

Clinical Features

(1) Lack of emotional response. Withdrawal and preoccupation.
(2) Silence and refusal to communicate (in some autistic children speech may not develop).
(3) The child does not play but may make up his own words and perform meaningless activities.

Management and treatment

The cause of this condition is unknown. Treatment may include tranquillisers, education, behaviour modifications and psycho-therapy. The autistic child benefits from a one to one relationship to stimulate communication and learning.

Mental disorders in adolescence

The psychiatric disorders of young adults may show in adoles-cence but the symptoms may reflect the behaviour of younger children.

Neurotic disorders

Free-floating anxiety, depression, phobias, hysterical reactions, bed-wetting, stomach upsets and tics may feature in adolescent psychiatry. Other patients may be aggressive or promiscuous and have a history of appearances in Juvenile Courts for truancy, stealing, damage to property, drug offences and lying.

Psychotic disorders

Schizophrenia may commonly appear following puberty. It may be slow to develop with vague behaviour which reflects an apparent laziness, loss of interest, day dreaming, falling-off in school work and so on, or it may have an acute onset. Diagnosis may be difficult and a period of observation is usually necessary before the illness is confirmed. Other psychotic conditions may include mania and depression.

Management of children and adolescents

Some disturbed children and adolescents may have a background of unhappy homes and parental neglect. Others may have been brought up in a materialistic background which lacked parental interest and understanding of their emotional needs.

The management of the variety of problems associated with the young persons may involve a variety of agencies and approaches:

1 Child guidance clinics. These clinics are run by the hospital service or as part of the school health service. Such clinics are usually staffed by a psychologist, a psychiatrist and a social worker. The child's problems are investigated and this may include a psychological assessment and social report on home background, school progress, and so on. Treatment may be aimed at improving parental difficulties, reassuring the family, modifying the child's environment or providing play therapy.

2 Children's psychiatric wards. Special wards may be provided in a psychiatric unit or children's hospital. The ward activities will need to be planned to cater for age and sex differences. A wide variety of games and activities are essential to absorb energies and prevent boredom. Occupational and educational therapy is important and provides opportunities for observation and outlets for constructive activity.

3 Adolescent units. Special adolescent units are now a feature in the management of adolescent problems. These units are small (usually 10–15 beds) and usually contain games rooms, a workshop, treatment rooms, single bedrooms and a classroom. A teacher is employed to ensure continuation of the young person's education.

Such units are proving to be valuable in the management of behaviour problems, and the treatments available may include psychotherapy, play therapy, work therapy, family therapy and drug therapy (e.g. tranquillisers). The treatment team normally includes a psychiatrist, psychologist, occupational therapist (or work instructor), social worker, and nursing staff.

Nursing care

Young children
The nurse should:
1 Reassure the child, and give support.
2 Encourage parents to visit and introduce them to the unit.
3 Act as parent substitute by showing interest, playing games, reading stories, giving affection and so on.
4 Provide outlets for energies, education and expression.
5 Discourage rule-breaking, disobedience, and other undesirable behaviour. The nurse should reward and approve good behaviour but be prepared to withdraw some privileges when persistent disobedience and rule-breaking occur.
6 Deal with child interactions such as quarrelling.
7 Comfort children during periods of distress.

Adolescents
The nurse should:
1 Develop an understanding, helpful and supporting relationship.
2 Promote self-esteem and combat rejection and feelings of insecurity.
3 Show interest in the adolescent as a person and be prepared to listen to his point of view.
4 Encourage the patient to relate with his peer group.
5 Develop active programmes for both indoor and outdoor activities.
6 Help with education and career ambitions.
7 Develop and teach social skills which will improve confidence e.g. dancing, debates, theatre and so on.
8 Promote personal hygiene and give tactful advice and help with cosmetics, fashion styles and so on.

9 Encourage self-help and participation in ward chores.

10 Encourage contact with family – gentle reminders to write home are often necessary.

11 Be fair with discipline and reward good behaviour.

28
Psychosomatic Disorders

Psychosomatic disorders are physical diseases which have an emotional element in their cause and development. The nature of these disorders can best be appreciated only when the patient's emotional disturbances (*Psycho*) are investigated along with the physical causes (*Soma*).

The patient's symptoms tend to be episodic, and each breakdown in the physical state may be brought about by an emotional crisis.

Many theories have been put forward to explain how organic disease may result from stress. It is generally accepted that since emotional factors can produce transient physical changes, (e.g., blushing, vomiting, diarrhoea, rapid pulse and so on), they may also produce longer lasting disturbances and chronic physical changes in body tissue.

Observations based on adrenocortical response to physical and emotional situations producing stress show how extreme cold, injury, subjection to anaesthesia and experiences such as taking exams, going for interview or awaiting surgery, are all accompanied by a rise in 17-hydroxycorticoid output.

Observational evidence by Wolf and Wolf (1947) on a patient 'Tom' who had a gastric fistula revealed how emotional changes influenced gastric functions. When the subject was angry his stomach lining was red and there were increased contractions and hydrochloric acid output. When the same subject was depressed or frightened the stomach lining was pale and there were decreased contractions and hydrochloric acid output.

Psychosomatic sufferers may show a particular type of personality (pre-morbid personality) which features traits such as anxiety, conscientiousness, ambition, rigidity and stubbornness.

Emotional stress brings about physiological changes through the autonomic and endocrine systems. Therefore, psychosomatic diseases tend to be associated with the cardiovascular system, the endocrine system, the gastro-intestinal tract and the skin. Some examples of psychosomatic diseases are given below.

Psychological asthma

Clinical features

The patient is often a child or young person and attacks may be associated with family disharmony or disappointment. Spasms of the smooth muscle of the bronchioles bring sudden attacks of dyspnoea with laboured and wheezy breathing. Attacks may last from a few minutes to hours or even days.

Differential diagnosis

Distinguish from other causes of asthma such as allergy or infection.

Complications

Status asthmaticus, bronchitis and heart failure may occur.

Management and treatment

(1) Psychotherapy for support, understanding and family rehabilitation. Hypnosis to relieve attacks.
(2) Bronchial dilators to relieve acute attacks (e.g. drugs such as beta$_2$ adrenoceptor stimulants).
(3) Breathing excercises to prevent chest deformity and faulty posture.
(4) Physical nursing care.

Peptic ulcers

Peptic ulceration can occur at any age and it may affect the stomach or duodenum. Most cases tend to become chronic and relapses with remissions is the usual course.

Clinical features

Epigastric pain related to meals, coming on just before a meal or after a meal. The pain is a burning sensation and is relieved by food and vomiting. The patient may suffer from nausea, insomnia and loss of weight.

Diagnosis

(1) Barium meal in preparation for an X-ray examination.
(2) Gastroscopic examination and fractional test meal.

Management and treatment

(1) Rest and physical nursing care.
(2) Psychotherapy.
(3) Drug therapy. (i) Diazepam (Valium) to sedate and relax. (ii) Drugs to relieve symptoms, e.g. antacids and anticholinergics. (iii) Histamine H$_2$ blockers such as cimetidine (Tagamet) 200 mg three times daily and 400 mg at bedtime is proving effective, or the alternative ranitidine 150 mg twice daily.
(4) Attention to diet – a non-irritating gastric diet may be helpful.
(5) Encouragement to stop smoking.
(6) Surgery (in some cases). This may be recommended for delayed healing ulcers and obstruction.

Complications

Haemorrhage, perforation and pyloric stenosis.

Ulcerative colitis

This condition causes severe inflammation and ulceration of the colon and rectum.

Clinical features

(1) Episodic attacks of diarrhoea with blood and mucus stools.
(2) Abdominal pain (colic type), loss of weight, insomnia and anaemia.

Diagnosis

(1) Sigmoidoscopy.
(2) Abdominal X-ray.
(3) Rectal biopsy and barium enema.

Management and treatment

(1) Rest and physical nursing care.
(2) Psychotherapy and tranquillisers (e.g. diazepam).
(3) Correction of dehydration and electrolyte deficiencies.
(4) Drugs. (i) Codeine Phosphate 30–60 mg six hourly to relieve diarrhoea. (ii) Anti-inflammatory drugs such as corticosteroids These may be given systemically (e.g. prednisone) or locally (e.g. prednisolone enemas).

(5) Surgery (in some cases). This may be necessary for chronic cases which do not respond to medical treatment. A procto-colectomy with a permanent ileostomy is usually necessary.
(6) Diet. Diet is important in the management of ulcerative colitis. A low residue diet with extra fluid is recommended to avoid colonic irritation.

Hypertension

Essential hypertension may be present for many years without causing many symptoms. With the permanently raised pressure, however, symptoms begin to appear and include: headaches, epistaxis, giddiness, buzzing ears and raised B/P.

Complications

Coronary Thrombosis, congestive heart failure, angina and cerebral haemorrhage (stroke).

Management and treatment

(1) Rest and physical nursing care.
(2) Psychotherapy and reassurance.
(3) Drugs. (i) A thiazide or similar diuretic. (ii) A beta adrenocep-tor blocker such as atenolol (Tenormin). (iii) A vasodilator such as hydralazine or prazosin. (iv) Methyldopa (Aldomet).
(4) Reduction in weight if obese, salt-restricted diet.
(5) Blood pressure recorded and charted twice daily.
(6) Rehabilitation to avoid stress and emotional upset. It may be necessary to adjust and lead a quieter life.
(7) Follow-up with family practitioner and checks on blood pressure.
(8) Avoidance of cigarette smoking.
(9) Monitor diuretic effects by weighing daily and check intake and output of fluids.

Thyrotoxicosis

This condition is produced by an excessive secretion of thyroid hormone (thyroxine). The cause is unknown but sometimes it may follow a severe emotional stress. The basal metabolic rate is raised.

Clinical features

(1) Onset may be rapid or insidious.

(2) Loss of weight and fatigue.
(3) Increased appetite, sweating and rapid irregular heart rate.
(4) Prominence of the eyes (exophthalmos).
(5) Fine tremor of tongue and fingers.
(6) Insomnia.
(7) Thyroid gland may be enlarged (goitre).
(8) Mental symptoms may include: irritability, anxiety, euphoria, over-activity, distractibility and delirium.

Diagnosis

Measurements of serum thyroxine and triiodothyronine levels, and thyroid hormone binding proteins.

Management and treatment

(1) Rest and full nursing care. Strategies for the nursing care plan should be designed following a detailed assessment which takes cognisance of common problems such as loss of weight, insomnia, restlessness, sweating, anxiety, overactivity and irritability.
(2) Psychotherapy, support and reassurance.
(3) Drugs. (i) Sedatives – chlorpromazine and diazepam (ii) Antithyroid drugs such as neo-mercazole (Carbimazole) 30 mg daily in divided doses.
(4) Radioactive iodine.
(5) Surgery and removal of 95 per cent of the gland.

Migraine

Migraine is characterised by periodic attacks of headaches which are often associated with eye disturbances and vomiting. The attacks are usually related to emotional stress and may come on at relaxation when the stress is over.

Clinical features

(1) Symptoms such as paraesthesiae or weakness of one side of the body or sometimes numbness of both hands.
(2) Coloured lights or spot sensations before the eyes.
(3) Severe throbbing headache usually on one side of the head.
(4) The headache may be accompanied by sweating and vomiting.
(5) The attack may last from a few hours to several days.

(6) The patient may be weak and exhausted on termination of an attack.

Management and treatment

(1) Rest in bed in a darkened room.

(2) Drugs. (i) Mild tranquilliser e.g. diazepam 2 mg three times daily. (ii) Methysergide 1 – 2 mg three times daily (given in severe cases).

(3) Psychotherapy and reassurance. Any anxiety about the cause of headache must be relieved.

(4) Physical nursing care and attention.

29

The Institutionalised
Patient and Rehabilitation

Recognising institutional neurosis

The term 'institutional neurosis' is used to describe characteristic features found in long-stay psychiatric patients. These features are an addition to the patient's underlying illness and are recognised by the following behaviour:

(1) Apathy, obedience and submissiveness with loss of interest and initiative and lack of individuality.

(2) Fixed routine behaviour with the patient showing dependence rather than independence.

(3) Negative and insignificant impact on others with a tendency to dirtiness and untidiness.

Causes

It is generally believed that institutionalised features can occur in any person confined to an institution for long periods. In addition to the patient's illness, there are many factors which facilitate the development of this condition. The most important factor may be the hospital and the patient's reactions to it. It is the hospital which appears to influence the patient's outlook and way of life. Observers have noted that this influence can be negative on the patient's behaviour to such an extent that he becomes dependent. He has little ambition for himself other than to be as secure as possible; he is content to allow the hospital to provide for his needs, give him a home, feed and clothe him, occupy him and so on.

The inherent factors in the environment likely to encourage such a negative attitude may include:

1 **Hospital impact.** Hospitals are big and overpowering, patients may feel small, insecure, exposed and vulnerable. The patient's initial reaction may be to maintain his individuality, initiative, interests and hobbies and so on. But the hospital may make this difficult for him. Failure of the institution to allow him to retain his personal possessions, to prevent boredom, to encourage contact with the outside world, to allow freedom, to provide outlets for his interests, to develop his personality, to communicate

his views, to be involved in his recovery and so on, may encourage him to develop a trouble-free institutional way of life.

2 Staff attitudes. Research has shown that some nurses tend to prefer patients who are co-operative. Those who complain, question, demand or disobey are unpopular. By nature the nurse feels more secure if the patient needs her. She wants to do things for the patient rather than with the patient. She expects obedience from her patients and respect for her authority.

The nurse should adopt a positive attitude to her patient's recovery: he is ill but also an individual; he has interests, he can think for himself and be independent; he can plan and organise for himself; he may have loved ones at home; he is not a hopeless case. The alternative to this may be loss of initiative and dependence so that the nurse is left with a co-operative, but sadly, an apathetic, institutionalised patient. From now on she must do and the patient be content to receive.

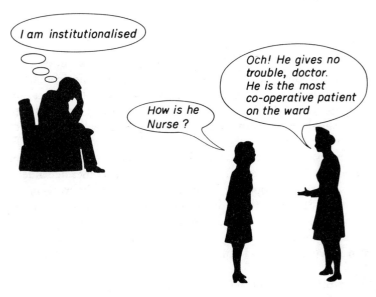

Fig. 29.1   Nursing means being troubled

Nursing care and management

Nursing approach. Initially, the nursing aim should be to prevent further institutionalisation and encourage remotivation in basic interests and self-help. At this level, much will depend on the individual nurse. It may be necessary for her to reappraise her own attitude to the patient. She may be used to the patient's way of life and may have learnt to accept it as being what is expected.

With this approach, the nurse is not neglecting the patient, she is caring for him but she may not help him to recover. In order to

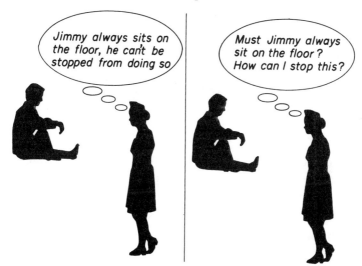

Fig. 29.2 Negative nursing   Positive nursing

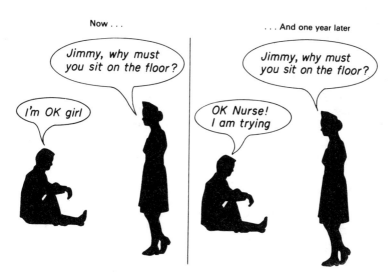

Fig. 29.3 The nurse must not give up

help the patient she must develop a therapeutic relationship with him and be prepared to inconvenience both herself and the patient to facilitate remotivation. It may be inconvenient for him to make his own bed if the nurse has always done this for him; but this is a positive inconvenience which must be encouraged. The nurse must show an interest in the patient's effort and help him to understand why she disapproves of his undesirable habits.

Encouraging the patient towards basic interests and self-help is not an easy task. It requires a great deal of nursing effort and patience. There will be numerous occasions when the nurse will feel frustrated because the patient is not responding. It is a constant struggle to remain positive but it is a vital one.

Rehabilitation

The objectives may be considered under four main headings.

1 *Self-help*

The rehabilitation plan should prepare the patient to function independently in society. He should learn to help himself over personal hygiene and dress, eating habits and domestic chores.

2 *Communication*

Some patients may require very little help with communications. Others, however, may have problems in this area. For example, they may avoid eye contact and verbal communication, their language may be foul or anti-social, they may not understand bus or train timetables and their knowledge of money may be limited. These basic skills are essential for personal function and may need inclusion in the recovery plan.

3 *Socialisation*

Institutionalised patients often lack the skills required to work and live with others. They may be loners with little idea about leisure activities or social obligations. Their behaviour may be undesirable and 'off-putting' to others and so on. The plan should introduce the patient to *social skill programmes* which will help him to learn and gain confidence for his social functioning.

> ### Unsocial Behaviour
>
> It is the small things which the public may find unacceptable, for example, dirtiness, untidiness, spitting, indecency, foul language, crazy talk, careless cigarette hygiene and fire hazards.

4 Work

Rehabilitating the patient to work is an important nursing objective. The patient may need to work for remuneration when he leaves hospital. He may need occupational training and help to find employment before he is discharged. In addition to learning motor skills involved in work training, the patient may need to learn how to cope in a factory or office setting.

Stages in rehabilitation

Rehabilitation may range from helping the patient to learn a simple task such as dressing or making a bed, to training in preparation for a job outside hospital. In preparing a plan of action, all aspects of the patient's life may need attention and the programme should reflect the training and experience necessary for each individual.

1 Assessment

An assessment of the patient's social, economic, physical and mental state should be made at the outset using the model outlined in Chapter 11. This should involve the ward team and at their meeting they should review the patient's treatment and discuss his interests, needs and wishes. Initial contact with his family should be made at this level.

2 Atmosphere

The right atmosphere is essential to give encouragement to both patients and staff. The staff should be enthusiastic and participate with the patient in rehabilitative activities. Progress should be recorded and reviewed regularly by the original assessment team. Upgrading of the patient's activities should be related to his progress. A change of ward environment may stimulate remotivation.

3 Involvement

The type of activities in which the patient is involved may include social skills, relearning, socialisation and preparation for resettlement and work. This may mean involvement at any stage in relearning about personal hygiene and domestic duties to the acquisition of new skills which will enable the patient to earn his living in society.

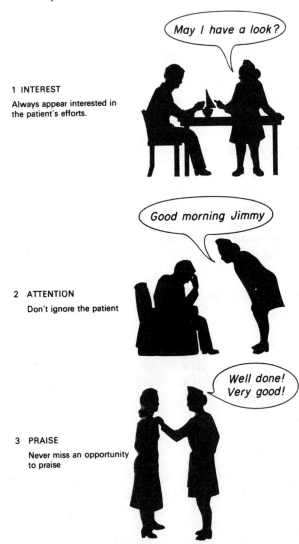

Fig. 29.4 The role of the nurse with the institutionalised patient

4 Resettlement

The later stages of rehabilitation must aim to prepare the patient for accommodation and work in the community. Self-care units are a feature of most hospitals which enable some patients to work outside hospital and live in on a part-time basis. Other patients may be discharged to hostels, flats, digs or other accommodation. All these approaches are helpful in preparing the patient to return to his family.

Relating resources to objectives

When planning a programme of activities, the nurse should relate involvement to the patient's needs and the rehabilitative objectives. Involvements should not be included merely for the sake of expediency.

It would not be sensible planning, e.g., to always include an untidy dependent female schizophrenic patient in recreational and industrial therapies but exclude her from educational, cookery,

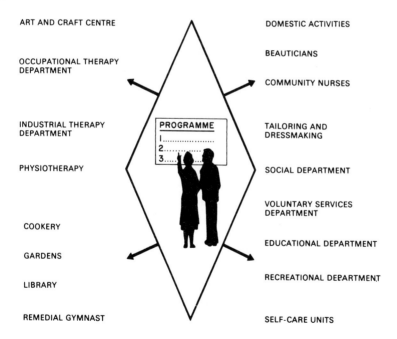

Fig. 29.5 Resources available to promote rehabilitation. The nurse should make the maximum use of resources to involve the patient in activities suitable for his stage of recovery and the rehabilitative objectives

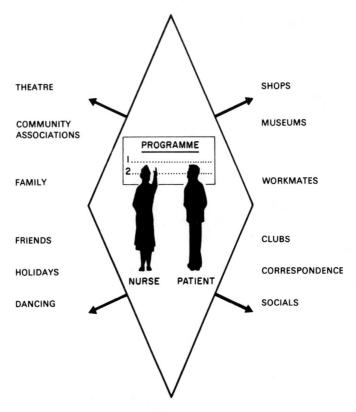

Fig. 29.6 Social rehabilitation. This should include opportunities for the development of interpersonal relationships and renewal of links with family, friends and social institutions

PERSONNEL	ACCOMMODATION
Patient's family	Self-care units
Social workers	Hostels
Community nurses	Flats and digs
Disablement Resettlement Officers	Private houses
Voluntary workers	Patient's home

Fig. 29.7 Resettlement. Though accommodation may be limited, there are many resources available to resettle and maintain the patient in the community

domestic, beauty and dressmaking classes. The hospital has a wide range of departments and personnel which practise activities suitable for all needs. In planning each patient's rehabilitation the nurse must balance the patient's involvements and include activities to meet the overall objectives. A good balanced programme for the aforementioned patient, e.g., should include all activities mentioned plus library activity, contact with voluntary workers, visits outside the hospitals and so on. The patient's response to activities should be evaluated continuously.

Note on social skills training

Many psychiatric patients, particularly the institutionalized, lack what may be called 'personal effectiveness'. Personally ineffectual people have difficulty meeting their social and material needs. Rather than taking an active part in their life circumstances, they are acted upon by others.

Being a personally effective person means that one is able to develop relationships with others and to tap and pursue common interests, individual goals and mutual satisfaction. It conveys the ability to understand, experience and appreciate other people and to make oneself better understood and appreciated. It also means being able to respect the rights of others and to assert one's own right. It involves love, tolerance and respect.

Social skills training can be successfully used to help long stay and other psychiatric patients to overcome their problems. The institutionalised patient can be helped to interact and communicate. *Aggressive patients* can be taught to express their anger and frustration in words. The nurse can be a key person in emphasising social skills learning by outlining broad objectives for each long stay patient's individual rehabilitation plan as follows:

1 To encourage a sense of awareness of self and others in social situations.

2 To identify, analyse, discriminate and practise specified social skills and to learn to recognise their use in different situations (e.g. friendship, concern, anger, joy, speaking, eye contact, pausing, sharing, listening, assertiveness, perceptual sensitivity, etc.).

Note on ward checklist

The Report of a Working Group '*Organisational and Management Problems of Mental Illness Hospitals*' (HMSO 1980), outlined a checklist for use at ward level. Such a checklist is useful for monitoring the care of long stay patients. A brief synopsis of the recommended check list includes a check on the ward environment, policies, goals, resources, staff activity, patient activity, food, clothing and so on. The reader should refer to the Report for specific details of the checklists which are essential to the care of the long stay mentally ill.

30

The Elderly Patient

Eighteen per cent of all admissions to psychiatric hospitals in the UK are over 65 years and 42 per cent of the beds are occupied by patients in this age category. With such a large number of elderly patients in hospital, the nurse may spend more time caring for elderly patients than other patient groups.

Staff attitudes

The elderly patient is an adult with wide experience of life; he may be a person who has brought up a family and lived through wars and economic depressions. The elderly person may also be a grandparent and he may live alone or have many friends.

Ironically, one notes frequent attitudes highlighted by comments such as 'in many ways they are like children', 'you must watch them', 'they need amusing', 'play along with them' etc. This attitude may be reflected in the nurse's relationship with the elderly patient and may be recognised by the absence of any spontaneous conversation.

It is important for the patients' self-esteem that they are cared for in a natural and spontaneous way. They should be treated as individuals and their quest for respect and indepencence should be met. This should be reflected in all aspects of the nurse's relationship with the patient, whether at a basic level, by allowing

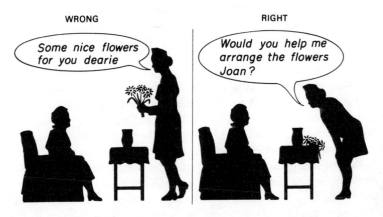

Fig. 30.1 Attitudes

the patient to eat with a knife and fork rather than a spoon, or at a more human level, by permitting the patients to form friendships and routines which matter to them.

Relationships

Initially there may be some difficulty in establishing a helping relationship with the elderly patient. Some may resent the dependence on nursing staff and become obstinate and critical of their efforts to help them. Some may be preoccupied with their bodily functions while others may be full of self-pity for their circumstances. On the other hand, some may be very pleasant and repeatedly thank the nurse for everything she does for them.

A nurse/patient relationship can bring about a marked improvement in the elderly person. The nurse can best establish this by showing an interest in the patient; she should never lose her temper but always show patience and understanding. The elderly patient will appreciate the nurse who considers his likes and dislikes. Old people may dislike having to ask for things, therefore, the nurse who can anticipate their needs can be very popular. The helpful nurse will develop a need in the patient to do things for himself. Such an approach will help to motivate the patient and add to his desire to feel useful and independent. The nurse should not expect too much from the patient and always be prepared to play down failures while boosting achievements.

Decline and the elderly person

It is an inescapable fact that the majority of elderly patients will show varying degrees of decline due to their age, illness or social circumstances. Another feature of the elderly patient is the way in which age, illness and social factors may interact. For example, an elderly woman may lose her husband and become depressed. She begins to neglect herself and may suffer the effects of malnutrition. She may be admitted to hospital with confusion or anaemia due to a combination of old age and social, physical and mental factors.

As we grow older our systems may function less efficiently and become more prone to disease. Joints may get stiff, breathlessness and coughing may be present, bladder and bowel disturbance is common, special senses may decline and so on. Social and economic factors may interact to speed up the decline or cause actual disease which might otherwise be prevented.

Effects of old age

System	Associated problems	Aggravating Factors*
Respiratory	Breathlessness Coughing Bronchitis Pneumonia	Poor housing
Circulatory	Hypertension Coronary disease Stroke	
Locomotor	Stiffness Rheumatoid arthritis Fractures	Social isolation Loneliness
Nutritional disturbance	Vitamin deficiencies Constipation Anaemia Lowered resistance	Poverty
Urinary	Bladder infections Incontinence	Cold weather Outside toilets
Nervous	Confusion Depression Dementia Tremors	Alcoholism Boredom Widowhood
Special senses	Deafness Poor eyesight	Physical disability

* When conducting a *social assessment* on the elderly patient the nurse should note factors which may aggravate the patient's condition on discharge from hospital. The appropriate *social intervention* will be a necessary part of rehabilitation and after care. For example, problems such as poor housing, social isolation, etc.

Community care

Ideally, the elderly person is best cared for in the familiar surrounding of his community and many services exist to encourage this and prevent hospitalisation. Services include:

Social Security. The old age pension goes some way towards helping the retired person to provide for his needs. Supplementary benefit may also be claimed (by persons who qualify) to help with expenses such as rent, heating and food. Most areas of the country also make concessions to the elderly for travel, public baths, fuel, entertainment and so on.

Accommodation. Most local authorities provide special accommodation (such as bungalows, flats and residential homes) for elderly persons. Warden-serviced blocks of flatlets are also provided by most cities.

Health and Social Services. The Health and Social Services provide a wide range of personnel and facilities for the elderly population. Services include social workers, district nurses, meals on wheels, laundry facilities, chiropody services, free prescriptions, dental and ophthalmic services. The *community psychiatric nurse* has a vital role to play in social intervention and after care.

Voluntary organisations. There are many voluntary groups which provide a wide range of services. They also visit old people in their homes, provide entertainments and run holiday homes.

Day hospitals. The day hospitals service is rapidly developing as a preventive measure against full-time hospitalisation. It is particularly beneficial for patients who are cared for at home but who may benefit from the investigations, treatment and social activities of the unit; for patients who require such support following discharge from hospital and to provide temporary relief for the families who care for the elderly at home.

Geriatric departments. The drift in the hospital care of the elderly patient is moving rapidly towards the concept of a special geriatric department. There are now over 200 such departments attached to hospitals throughout the UK and more are developing each year. These departments are designed and organised to facilitate the care, treatment and rehabilitation of elderly persons.

Structurally, the units are designed to facilitate patient mobility, to prevent accidents, to facilitate nursing care and observation and to promote rehabilitation. A team approach to care is the practice and includes the following personnel:

Immediate Members	Supporting Members
Doctors	General Practitioners
Nurses	Social workers
Remedial gymnasts	Community nurses
Physiotherapists	Voluntary workers
Occupational therapists	Hostel supervisors

The majority of geriatric departments have an admission unit where the patient is initially received and diagnosed. Early treatment, nursing care and rehabilitation are concurrent, with the latter developing at different stages until self-help and independence are reached.

Throughout the treatment process, strong links and close co-operation are maintained with community services to enable early discharge with short term readmission when necessary. Some may not recover sufficiently to leave hospital and will require long-term nursing care in a homely ward.

Factors involved in nursing the elderly

A Assessment
Many aspects are involved in the care of the elderly patient and the process should commence with an *assessment* of the patient under the following headings:

1 *Reasons for Admission.* Note the present reasons, past admissions and the patient's and family's perception and understanding of illness and admission.

2 *General Condition on Admission.* Observe the state of hair, teeth, skin, personal hygiene, marks, swellings, continence control, dressing, wounds, pain, colour, breathing, mobility, level of consciousness, orientation, co-operation, TPR and urine analysis.

3 *General Health History.* Any underlying diseases, allergies, handicaps, and so on.

4 *Daily Living Activities.* Assess dietary needs, breathing, bladder, bowels, sleep, mobility, aids, interests.

5 *Personality.* Level of social skills, motivation, dependence, independence, attitude to illness and hospitalization, ability to cope with stress, pain or insomnia, mood and personality traits (e.g. suspicion).

6 *Socio-Economic.* Occupation, source of income, marital state, dependants, home conditions, visiting problems, domestic arrangements while in hospital and potential problems on discharge. Role of District Nurse, Community Psychiatric Nurse or Social Worker.

7 *Risk Factors/Safety.* Assess risks of infection, pressure sores, accidents, drug side effects and confusion.

8 *Treatments — Investigations*
Refer to Medical Notes.

B Brief for guiding nursing care

Problem	Goal	Intervention	Evaluation
Sleep	Promote sleep coping resources	Attend to insomnia factors	Maintain sleep record Observe hypnotice effects
Diet	Diet education and training	Balanced diet Domestic rehabilitation Fluids	Record weight Food intake and fluid intake – output
Bowels	Promote regular bowel habits	Anticipate toilet needs Prevent constipation Investigate diarrhoea	Record bowel movements
Bladder	Promote regular habits	Anticipate needs Regular toileting	Record urinary output Is specimen needed?
Exercise	Maintain mobility	Daily exercises Physiotherapy	Note immobilising factors Are walking aids necessary?
Feet	Prevent immobility and discomfort	Correct footwear Chiropoly	Note foot abnormalities
Hands	Promote dexterity and cleanliness	Regular hygiene and manicure Exercise	Note tremors Will treatment increases dexterity?
Teeth	Maintain hygiene	Regular oral hygiene Denture care	Are dental appointments necessary?
Sight	Prevent perceptual errors and accidents	Facilitate shortsight Care of spectacles	Are optical appointments necessary? *Continued*

Problem	Goal	Intervention	Evaluation
Hearing	Promote orientation	Adapt communication modes to quality of hearing	Are aids necessary? Is there wax in ears?
Bathing	Promote cleanliness and comfort	Regular bath or shower	Does the patient wash properly? Observe for marks. Do nails need trimming?
Confusion	Prevent confusion Promote orientation	Reality orientation	Is confusion a risk factor?
Boredom	Promote interests and activities	Introduce to occupational/ social therapies	Note level of patient participation and rehabilitative effects
Routine	Promote self help and independence	Maintain a slow flexible routine	Does the patient understand the routine?
Accidents	Promote safety and prevent injury	Maintain a safe environment Eliminate accident risks	Is the patient prone to accidents or wandering?

Note on nursing care

The problems, goals and interventions outlined for the elderly patient are not definite. Patients who are bedridden will require much nursing help with oral hygiene, bed bathing, hairwashing, prevention of pressure sores, prevention of foot drop and so on. For procedural detail the reader should refer to a Nursing Procedures Book.

Note on reality orientation

Reality orientation programmes have much to offer in the supportive care of the elderly hospitalised patient. In essence, reality orientation is a method for communicating with elderly confused people in such a way that they are repeatedly supplied with information on their own whereabouts, the time of day, date, what is happening to them and their own and other people's identity. All staff involved with the patients must be consistent in their approach and adhere to the programme's objectives. Research has shown that this technique can improve elderly people's orientation and social behaviour (See Merchant and Saxby, 1981).

31

The Patient
and his Rights

Provisions for mental health legislation vary from one country to another, and from state to state in the USA. They all have general similarities and provide for the following.

Informal care

About 95 per cent of patients admitted to psychiatric hospitals receive care and treatment on an informal basis. The patient enters hospital of his own free will, cannot be compelled to take treatment without his consent, and retains the right to self-discharge. British legislation contains no provisions which authorise staff to lock an informal patient in a single room or detain him in a locked ward. The responsibilities of staff to an informal patient are the same as those of staff to a patient in a non-psychiatric hospital. However, caring staff in hospitals have a duty under Common Law to prevent patients coming to harm, such as suicidal patients, the elderly and confused or others at risk (see also Chapter 36).

Should an informal patient express a desire to leave hospital it may be difficult to tell whether it is a passing whim rather than a real wish. However, in cases where it is considered unwise to allow the patient to leave, staff must reassure the patient and persuade him to remain. Persuasion should not be excessive. If the patient persists he must either be allowed to leave, (by signing a Discharge Against Medical Advice form), or detained under compulsory powers.

Under English legislation an informal patient may be prevented from leaving hospital, if he is a danger to himself or others, by a Section 5(11) 72 hour detention report signed by the registered medical practitioner. The 1983 Mental Health Act (England and Wales) makes provisions under Section 5(4) for a nurse of the prescribed class to hold an informal patient for 6 hours (in Scotland it is for 2 hours; in Northern Ireland 6 hours has been recommended but is not yet law). An example of the form for a nurse's application under Section 5(4) is given below:

Section 5(4)

NURSE'S REPORT ON AN INFORMAL PATIENT

PART I

NAME OF PATIENT.............. Date of Admission ....

ADDRESS .... Time of Report ....

.... Time Holding power expires

....

PART II

1 I...

OF...

being a nurse of the prescribed class detain the patient named in Part I of this Report

2 I am of the opinion
   (a) that the patient is suffering from mental disorder to such a degree that it is necessary for his health and safety or for the protection of others for him to be immediately restrained from leaving the hospital and
   (b) that it is not practicable to secure the immediate attendance of a medical practitioner for the purpose of furnishing a Report under sub section 2 of this section.

3 My opinion based on the following nursing assessment ....

....

....

....

....

To .... Health and Social Services Board

Nurse's signature ....

Date ....

Formal care

A minority of psychiatric patients are cared for on a formal basis. This means that some other person or persons (usually a relative or a social worker and a doctor) has taken steps to enforce the patient's admission to hospital for treatment and care. The reason for such action may be that the patient cannot act in his own interests, is neglecting his mental health, or is a danger to the public.

The procedure for evoking a formal admission includes an application by the patient's relative or social worker and this must be supported by medical recommendations from a doctor or doctors who have examined the patient. There is usually more than one type of formal admission and they vary from a temporary emergency type to a more permanent detention period. In some cases the admission may be evoked from the courts. As formal admission interferes with the patient's civil rights, safeguards are built in to the legislation to protect the patient's rights concerning discharge, treatment, property, correspondence and so on.

Rights of formal patients and relatives

Staff have a duty to inform patients and relatives of their rights under Mental Health Legislation. Ideally the hospital administration should provide a leaflet for this purpose. Rights are considered under the following headings:

1 Detention and discharge

The detention period for formal patients is related to the type of order under which they are being detained. Detention periods may be specified for a short period or for much longer periods (see Mental Health Acts in Chapter 32).

Patients liable to long-term detention may seek their discharge from the Responsible Medical Officer (RMO) or from the hospital management. In some countries (UK), the legislation allows the patient's nearest relative powers to discharge.

Patients and relatives who are refused discharge requests have other avenues which they can explore. For example, they can appeal to judicial or semi-judicial bodies. These bodies are independent and can over-rule the doctor and administration by discharging the patient should they find in his favour. Independent review bodies exist in many countries but not all. Some examples are: the Mental Health Information Services, New York State; the Mental Health Review Tribunals in England, Wales and Northern Ireland; the Mental Welfare Commission in Scotland; the Mental Health Review Board, Ontario, Canada. In England, Scotland, Wales and Northern Ireland, patients detained through the courts can appeal against the sentence or apply for review to the Home Secretary or Secretary of State of the countries mentioned.

2 Property and affairs

The nature of some patients' mental disorder may make them incapable of managing their property and affairs. Most legislation permits the appointment of a receiver or guardian to be responsible for managing the patient's affairs. The receiver or curator controls will be specified by the protection court as the Judge directs. As soon as the patient is well enough to assume responsibilities again, the receiver will be disbanded. This procedure prevents the patient from squandering his assets or other people from taking advantage and frittering away his property and money.

3 Staff malpractices

Mental Health Legislation discourages offences against the patient by providing for punishment of those who commit them. For example, it is an offence under the Mental Health Act for England and Wales:
 (a) To ill-treat a patient.
 (b) For a male staff member to have sexual intercourse with a mentally disordered female.
 (c) To forge documents authorised in the Act.
 (d) To assist patients to abscond or to harbour absconded patients.

4 Wills and contracts

Legal capacity depends on a person's understanding of what he is doing and the effects of doing it. The important factor, therefore, is not whether the patient is formal or informal but whether his illness makes him legally incapable of performing the functions involved in making wills or entering contracts. A patient can make a valid will providing his illness does not interfere with his legal capacity, and patients who enter contracts before mental breakdown, or during a lucid interval in their illness, are party to the agreement even in later years.

The legal capacity for making a will is taken from a statement in the *Banks* v *Goodfellow* (1870) ruling as follows:
'He ought to be capable of making his will with an understanding of the nature of the business in which he is engaged, a recollection of the property he means to dispose of, or the persons who are the object of his bounty, and the manner in which it is to be distributed between them.'
The patient need only do this in simple terms.

Neither does it matter if the patient is deluded or hallucinated providing such symptoms do not interfere with his thinking in respect of the above statement. A medical opinion is usually necessary to establish whether the illness affects the patient's legal capacity.

When a patient makes a request to prepare a will the nurse should make an appointment for the patient's solicitor to visit him. In an emergency, the patient can make a will in the presence of two independent witnesses who should also sign in the presence of each other. Hospital administrators can be witnesses, but not nurses who might, unwittingly, influence their patients.

The English Administration of Justices Act (1969) ruled that if a patient is deemed incapable of making a will and the rule for inheritance on intestacy is inadequate, then the Court of Protection is empowered to make a will on the patient's behalf.

5 Divorce

Long-term patients can be sued for divorce by their spouse following a period of continuous hospitalisation for mental illness, usually two years (on the grounds of irretrievable breakdown – 1973 Matrimonial Causes Act). It is the duty of nursing staff to help to reassure such patients in coming to terms with the realities of their situation.

The hospital has a duty to help the patient to obtain whatever advice or assistance he may need.

6 Marriage

A marriage may be void if at the time of the ceremony the bride or groom could not understand the contract because of mental disorder. A marriage may be annulled if either party was suffering from a mental disorder at the time of the ceremony (whether continuously or intermittently), which rendered them unfit for marriage.

7 Occupation

A patient who has been in employment for some time, (52 weeks for full-time employment) may appeal to an Industrial Review Tribunal for unfair dismissal if his employer terminated his contract because of his illness or hospitalisation. Absence from work because of ill-health can be a good reason for dismissal providing that in all the circumstances the employer was reasonable in treating it as such.

8 Income

Whether a patient will receive money from his employer during hospitalisation will depend on the terms of his contract. Social security benefit is not reduced for the first eight weeks but from weeks 8—52 it is reduced. After 52 weeks the patient only receives benefit at pocket money level but if he has dependents the remainder can be paid directly to them.

9 Leave of absence

The Responsible Medical Officer may grant leave of absence either conditional or unconditional. The leave may be specified, e.g. Monday to Friday, or it may be open-ended.

The patient's progress during leave of absence will provide good feedback on his treatment and recovery. Before going on leave, the nurse should ensure that the patient and relative are informed about medication, nursing requirements, and date of return. The relatives should be further reassured that should the patient regress they may return him to hospital before leave expires.

On return from leave the nurse should talk with the patient and his relatives for feedback purposes.

10 Absence without leave (AWOL)

Some patients may occasionally abscond from the hospital where they are being detained. On suspecting a patient to be absent the nurse should check the ward to ensure that the patient is not still on the premises. Once satisfied that the patient is AWOL the nursing administration and ward doctor should be informed. The nursing officer will require a description of the patient, type of clothing worn, when last seen, treatment and so on.

Should an informal patient go absent without leave, the nurse has a Common Law duty to make follow-up enquiries regarding his safety. Although the informal patient cannot be returned, if he refuses to do so, the nurse should ensure that he has come to no harm. After all, it is possible that he may have wandered in a confused state or have been involved in a road traffic accident and so on.

11 Consent to treatment

It is generally accepted that no one may wilfully interfere with the body of another person without their consent and anyone who does so is liable to an action for damages. In the case of persons under 16 years, the consent of parent or guardian is necessary.

What is consent? Consent is not simply a matter of obtaining a signature on a form. It is generally accepted that for consent to be valid it must be a free and informed consent. Ambiguity in consent should be avoided by ensuring that the patient is given all the relevant information relating to the proposed treatment. In so far as is possible, consent should include an understanding of the treatment including any likely complications and adverse side effects. Obtaining the patient's consent is the responsibility of the doctor and any doubts expressed by the patient should be discussed with the RMO otherwise the consent may be invalidated.

In mental disorder some patients may be unable to give a full and informed consent. Also the law surrounding consent to treatment by the mentally disordered is uncertain and controversial. Some patients may appear backward due to mental disorder but this is no reason for assuming that they cannot give a valid consent. Also, if the patient appears to have difficulty understanding what the treatment involves, it is best to assume that he has not consented.

It is the duty of hospital managers to inform patients of thier rights in respect of consent including their right to refuse or ask for a second opinion.

In the case of treatment by drugs it is usually sufficient to obtain oral consent but in all requests for consent the nurse should relate to the guidelines and standardised forms in current use by her Health Authority. In the final analysis, unauthorised treatment can result in an action for damages and the doctor and hospital management will be held responsible.

The reader should refer to Chapter 32 and sections 56–64 of the Mental Health Act 1983 (England and Wales) for the current legal aspect of consent to treatment.

12 *Accidents*

Patients who receive injuries in hospital may claim damages against the hospital management. The nurse should be constantly aware of factors which may cause injury to patients and be vigilant in prevention at all times. However, accidents will happen and it is essential that the full circumstances regarding the accident are recorded in a written form, (including statements from witnesses and follow-up medical and nursing attention). In most cases the hospital will accept responsibility for any claims resulting from accidents but this does not rule out a case being brought against a staff member who injures a patient due to negligence or incompetence.

13 Private medical examination

Under some mental health acts (such as that for Northern Ireland), a patient who is liable to detention in hospital is permitted to have a doctor of his own choice, or that of his nearest relative, to visit, examine him in private and advise him about his rights to appeal or the right of his nearest relative to order his discharge.

14 Human dignity

Some aspects of treatment and hospitalisation may threaten the patient's dignity. All patients have the right to be recognised and consulted about treatments and procedures which involve them. The nurse must respect the patient as a person, promote his self-esteem, ensure comfort and protect him from embarrassment and ridicule insofar as is possible.

15 Voting rights of patients

British Common Law holds that 'idiots' and persons of unsound mind cannot vote or stand for election to public office. This now bears no relation to the 1983 Mental Health Act. Some problems may arise for patients who are in hospital on the qualifying date because the Representation of the Peoples Act (1949) disenfranchises people in establishments maintained wholly or mainly for those suffering from mental disorders. However, the British Government supports the recommendation of the Speakers Conference (1974) that patients in mental hospitals should be treated similarly to those in general hospitals.

Unless detained on a section, all in-patients, including those admitted informally, are eligible to vote. Patients wishing to vote should complete a 'patient's declaration' (schedule 2 1982 Mental Health Act Amendment) which, if accepted by the Registration Officer, will ensure that their name is included on the electoral register. Patients may not give the hospital as their address, however, and may not be helped to complete their registration form.

Investigation agencies

A number of agencies have been developed for the purpose of monitoring the services and/or investigating individual complaints. These are:

1 Hospital Advisory Service

This independent advisory service was established in 1969 to advise the Secretary of State on standards of care and management practices in individual hospitals in England and Wales. The service is composed of doctors, nurses, administrators and others, who visit hospitals for inspection, produce a report and make recommendations.

2 Health Service Commissioners

These are appointed with powers to investigate individual complaints referred to them. If a patient is unable to act for himself, a complaint may be made to the Commissioner on his behalf by a person or organisation suitable to represent him. Members of the hospital staff can submit complaints on behalf of patients who are unable to act for themselves (see also Chapter 36).

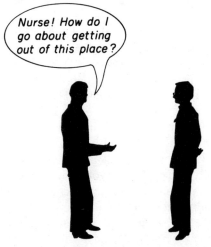

The nurse has a duty to inform the patient of his rights

Fig. 31.1 The detained patient

3 Mental Health Act Commission

(a) Section 120 of the Mental Health Act 1983 states that the Secretary of State shall make arrangements for persons authorised by him to investigate any complaint made by a person who is or has been detained under the Act and which he considers has not been satisfactorily dealt with by the managers of the hospital.

(b) Section 121 of the 1983 Act states that the Secretary of State shall direct the Mental Health Act Commission to keep under review the care and treatment of patients in hospitals not liable to be detained under the Mental Health Act. The Commission shall also review any decision to withold a postal packet to a patient detained in a Special Hospital.

32

Mental Health Laws of Great Britain and the Republic of Ireland

The Mental Health Act 1983 (England and Wales)

Mental disorder
The Mental Health Act 1983 defines this as mental illness, arrested or incomplete development of the mind, psychopathic disorder, and any other disorder or disability of the mind.

There are four types of disorder within Section 1 of the Act. The Act defines severe mental impairment, mental impairment and psychopathic disorder. Mental illness is not defined.

Severe mental impairment is defined as a state of arrested or incomplete development of mind which includes severe impairment of intelligence and social functioning and is associated with abnormally aggressive or seriously irresponsible conduct on the part of the person concerned.

Mental impairment is defined as a state of arrested or incomplete development of mind (not amounting to severe mental impairment) which includes significant impairment of intelligence and social functioning and is associated with abnormally aggressive or seriously irresponsible conduct on the part of the person concerned.

Psychopathic disorder is defined as a persistent disorder or disability of mind (whether or not including significant impairment of intelligence) which results in abnormally aggressive or seriously irresponsible conduct on the part of the person concerned.

Informal admission

Reference: *Section 131*
An informal patient enters hospital on the advice of his doctor for care and treatment. This is a voluntary act. The patient has the

right to refuse treatment and to discharge himself (see page 218). He retains his legal rights, including the right to vote (see page 225). Ninety four per cent of patients in mental institutions are informal.

Formal admission

Admission for assessment

(a) Reference: *Section 2*
This requires an application for admission to detain a patient in a hospital for assessment (or for assessment followed by treatment). Application is made by the nearest relative or an approved social worker and supported by two medical recommendations.

The Assessment period is for 28 days.

(b) Reference: *Section 4*
This is an emergency application for admission for assessment. Application is by the nearest relative or an approved social worker supported by one medical recommendation.

The Assessment period is for 72 hours. Fifty five per cent of formal admissions are 72 hour emergencies.

Admimission for treatment

Reference: *Section 3*
An application is completed by the nearest relative or an approved social worker supported by two medical recommendations (under certain circumstances both medical recommendations may be given by doctors on the hospital staff— *Section 12*).

Initially detention is for six months, renewable for six months and then renewable for one year.

Note on applications

Reference: *Section 13*
(a) Before making an application the approved social worker shall assess the appropriateness for admission.

(b) Hospital managers shall request a social report in cases where the application is made out by the nearest relative (excluding emergency admission).

Patients already in hospital

Reference: *Section 5*
The medical practitioner in charge of the treatment of an informal patient (or another nominated medical practitioner) completes a Report which detains the patient for 72 hours.

Nurse's role. If it appears to a nurse of the prescribed class (prescribed by an order from the Secretary of State) that an informal patient requires immediate restraint from leaving the ward and that it is not practicable to secure the immediate attendance of a doctor to complete the Detention Report, the nurse must record the fact in writing to the hospital managers and may hold the patient for up to six hours from the time of recording or until the earlier arrival of the doctor (Section 5(4)).

Admission of patients concerned in criminal proceedings

(a) Reference: *Section 37*
An admission to hospital from the courts of an offender with mental disorder. Medical evidence must be presented to the courts for an offender to be admitted to hospital.

(b) Reference: *Section 41*
This applies a restriction order to the court admission. The Secretary of State may refer the case of a restricted patient to the Mental Health Review Tribunal at any time.

Transfer of a mentally disordered person from prison to hospital

(a) Reference: *Section 47*
Transfer of a prisoner to hospital without a restriction order.

(b) References: *Sections 49–50*
Transfer of a prisoner to hospital with restrictions.

Remand admissions

(a) Reference: *Section 35*
A Crown Court or Magistrates Court may remand an accused person to hospital for a Report on his mental state.

(b) Reference: *Section 36*
A Crown Court may remand an accused person to hospital for treatment if satisfied on the evidence of two medical practitioners

that he is suffering from mental illness or severe mental impairment.

Interim hospital orders

Reference: *Section 38*
An interim hospital order may be applied to a convicted person for a period of twelve weeks, renewable for periods of 28 days. No such order shall continue for more than 6 months.

Admission to a place of safety

Reference: Section 135
A mentally disordered person may be removed to a place of safety because of ill treatment or neglect.
The detention period is for 72 hours.

Police admission

Reference: *Section 136*
A mentally disordered person found in a public place and behaving in a manner which is a danger to himself or others may be removed to a place of safety by any police constable.
The detention period is 72 hours.

Leave of absence

Reference: *Section 17*
Leave of absence may be granted to a detained patient (excluding restricted patients) by the Responsible Medical Officer either conditionally or unconditionally.
The maximum leave period is 6 months.

Absent without leave (AWOL)

Reference: *Section 18*
An absconding patient may be returned by any police constable, any officer of hospital staff or any approved social worker.

Correspondence of patients

Reference: *Section 134*
(1) Letters from detained patients may be witheld from the Post Office at the request of the addressee.

(2) Patients in Special Hospitals may have their mail censored by the hospital managers.

(3) Letters to the following are excluded from censorship: any Minister or Member of Parliament of either House, Court of Protection, Commissioner of Complaints, Mental Health Review Tribunal, Health Authority, Hospital Managers, Patient's Legal Advisor and European Commission or Court of Human Rights.

(4) When a patient's letter is withheld the managers shall keep a record and inform the patient within 7 days.

Discharge

Reference: *Section 23*

Powers of discharge are granted to the Responsible Medical Officer, Hospital Managers, the Mental Health Review Tribunal and the nearest relative in respect of detained and assessment patients. The nearest relative must give 72 hours notice in writing and if barred from exercising their power they may appeal to the Mental Health Review Tribunal.

The nearest relative must be given 7 days notice of intention to discharge a detained patient.

Mental Health Review Tribunals

References: *Sections 65 – 79*

Constitution. Tribunals are appointed by the Lord Chancellor. They have a minimum of 3 members, i.e. a legal member, a medical member and a social administrative person.

Powers. Tribunals may discharge, re-classify, transfer or grant leave to patients detained for assessment or treatment. Under certain circumstances tribunals may absolutely or conditionally discharge restricted patients.

Applications. (1) Assessment patients may apply within the first 14 days. (2) Treatment patients may apply within the first six months and within 28 days following renewals. (3) Hospital managers may refer patients after a 3 year period. (4) Nearest relatives may apply on behalf of patients.

Court of Protection

Reference: *Section 93*

The Court of Protection may appoint a receiver to manage the property and affairs of persons with mental disability.

Consent to treatment

References: *Sections 56–64*
(a) A patient shall not be given certain treatments (e.g. psycho-surgery) without his consent. A medical practitioner (not being the Responsible Medical Officer) must also consult two other persons professionally concerned with the patient's treatment and certify to the treatment in writing. One of the latter persons shall be a nurse.
(b) A medicine may not be administered to a patient if 3 months have elapsed since medicine was first administered unless the patient has consented and a medical officer certifies to this consent in writing.

In cases where the patient is not capable of consenting a medical practitioner (not being the Responsible Medical Officer) shall consult two other persons professionally concerned with the patient's treatment and certify in writing that the treatment should be given.

N.B. Provisions in (a) and (b) also apply to informal patients.

(c) The constraints relating to consent shall not apply to urgent treatment. Any treatment (not being irreversible or hazardous) may be given if it is immediately necessary to save life, alleviate serious suffering or prevent serious deterioration in the patient's condition or is immediately necessary to prevent a patient from behaving violently or being a danger to himself or to others.

Code of practice

Reference: *Section 118*
A code of practice will be prepared by the Secretary of State for the guidance of medical practitioners, managers and staff in relation to admissions and treatments.

Information to detained patients

Reference: *Section 132*
Hospital managers shall inform detained patients of their rights.

Mental Health Act Commission

Reference: *Section 121*
A Mental Health Act Commission has been established by the Secretary of State to perform on his behalf the following:

1 Appoint medical practitioners for the purposes of consent.
2 Review patients' treatments.
3 Visit detained patients, interview patients, review detention and generally protect detained patients' rights.
4 Investigate complaints and review decisions to withold patients' letters.

Protection of staff

Reference: *Section 139*
Staff are protected from legal proceedings arising from their work unless they act in bad faith or without reasonable care. Civil or criminal proceedings shall not be instigated without the consent of the Director of Public Prosecutions.

2 The 1961 Mental Health Act (Northern Ireland)

This act delegates powers to the Ministry and Area Boards to make provisions for the prevention, diagnosis, treatment, care supervision, training, occupation and co-ordination of services for persons with a mental disorder.

Section 6

This allows for informal use of the services.

Section 7

This defines mental disorder as mental illness, arrested or incomplete development of the mind, or any other disorder or disability of the mind. Mental handicap is established on the basis of intelligence and social functioning ability.

Formal admissions

Sections 12—14

These provide for a patient to be admitted and detained for 21 days on completion of an application by the nearest relative or social worker and a medical recommendation by the family practitioner (Form 2). The admitting doctor must examine the patient and complete Form 5 (Section 18).

Section 15

This provides for an emergency admission with a seven day detention period on the completion of an application by any relative or social worker and a medical recommendation by the family doctor (Form 3).

Section 16

This provides for the detention of an informal patient for three days (Form 4).

Section 19

This provides for the extention of the 21 and 7 day detention periods to six months (Form 6).

Section 32

This provides for the extension of the six month detention period for one further year (Form 8), and thereafter for two year periods (Form 9).

Section 48

This provides for court admission without restriction, (similar to S37 England and Wales).

Section 53

This provides for court admission with restrictions, (see S41 England and Wales).

Section 105

This deals with removal to a place of safety, (see S135 England and Wales).

Section 106

This deals with police admission, (see S136 England and Wales).

Section 25

This deals with patients' mail. Provisions are the same as S134 in the England and Wales Act, except that mail is not liable to censorship.

Section 29

This deals with leave of absence, (similar to S17 England and Wales).

Section 30

This deals with absence without leave, (similar to S18 England and Wales).

Sections 76–79

These make provisions for the Mental Health Review Tribunal. One Tribunal exists for the province and the members are appointed by the Lord Chief Justice. Otherwise, the terms are the same as outlined for the England and Wales Act.

Section 35

This makes provisions for discharge, (similar to S23 England and Wales).

Section 73

This makes provisions for the management of the property and affairs of mentally disordered persons. It is similar to the Court of Protection in the England and Wales Act, but uses the Department of Affairs for Mental Patients.

Review of the Northern Ireland Mental Health Act 1981

Reference: *Northern Ireland Review Committee on Mental Health Legislation*, HMSO (1981)

This review proposes the following amendments to the 1961 Act:

1 An innovative definition for Mental Illness
2 A single admission procedure for a 7 day assessment renewable for a further 7 days
3 Detention periods for treatment to read 6 months, renewable for 6 months, renewable for 1 year and yearly thereafter
4 Power to allow a nursing officer to hold an informal patient for 6 hours
5 A Mental Health Act Commission to be established
6 Special Care to be reclassified as Mental Handicap

3 The Mental Health Act (Scotland) 1960

This Act repealed the Scottish Lunacy and Mental Deficiency Acts, abolished the Board of Control and established the Mental Welfare Commission for Scotland.

Constitution of the Mental Welfare Commission (Section 2)

This states that the Commission will consist of a minimum of seven members to include at least three medical members, one legal member and at least one woman member. Four commissioners (including one medical member) shall constitute a quorum.

Functions and duties of the Commission

The Commission exercises protective functions for mentally disordered people who are incapable of protecting their persons or their interests and who are liable to detention. It does this by:

(a) Making enquiries regarding cases of ill-treatment, deficient care or treatment, improper detention and loss of patients' property.
(b) Making regular visits to patients liable to be detained in hospital. This may include interviewing and examining patients in private during visits.
(c) Discharging patients in appropriate cases.

Section 6

This defines mental disorder as mental illness or mental deficiency, however caused or manifested.

Section 23 (1)

This defines patients liable to detention as persons suffering from any mental disorder that requires or is susceptible to treatment. It states that no person over 21 years shall be admitted (except in an emergency) unless he is agressive or shows seriously irresponsible conduct.

Section 23 (3)

This provides for informal use of the service.

Section 24

This provides for a compulsory admission with a detention period of one year, renewable for one further year and then for two yearly periods (S39 duration of detention). An application is completed by either the nearest relative or the mental welfare officer (S26) and supported by two medical recommendations (one from a psychiatrist and one from the family doctor).

Application approval by the Sheriff

Applications for admission must be submitted to the Sheriff for his approval (S28).

Functions of the Sheriff. The Sheriff considers applications, approves them and hears objections from the nearest relative.

Effect of applications. An application approved by the Sheriff is sufficient for the patient's removal to hospital within seven days. The admitting hospital management must inform the Mental Welfare Commission of the admission within seven days of the patient's arrival in hospital.

Section 31

This provides for an emergency admission with a seven day detention period. A statement of consent from a relative or mental health officer supported by one medical recommendation is required.

Section 32

This states that an application for admission or an emergency recommendation may be made to detain an informal patient.

Section 54

This makes provision for a court to commit a mentally disordered offender to hospital instead of remanding him in custody. Medical evidence is necessary.

Section 55

This makes provision for the admission of a mentally disordered person from a High Court or a Sheriff's Court without restrictions, (the requirements are the same as for Section 37 England and Wales Act).

Section 60

This provides for a court admission with restrictions which may be without limit of time or time as specified in the order. Patients admitted in this way can only be granted leave or discharge by the Secretary of State for Scotland. Requirements for this admission are similar to those in S41 England and Wales Act.

Section 66

This provides for the transfer of a mentally disordered person from prison to hospital. (It may be accompanied by a restriction order S60.)

Section 89

This states that the Secretary of State for Scotland shall provide state hospitals for detained persons who require treatment under special security conditions.

Section 103

This makes provision for the removal of a mentally disordered person to a place of safety for 72 hours.

Section 104

This makes provision for a police constable to remove a mentally disordered person from a public place to a place of safety for 72 hours.

Discharge (Section 43)

This states that a detained patient may be discharged by any of the following: the Responsible Medical Officer, the Mental Welfare

Commission, the Sheriff (under a Sheriff's appeal Section 39), the Hospital Management (with the RMO's consent Section 43 (5)) or the nearerst relative (who must give seven days' notice in writing). The RMO may furnish a report to the hospital management advising against the nearest relative's request to discharge. Such a report prevents the relative's order of discharge from taking effect. The nearest relative may not exercise his/her right for a period of six months, but can appeal to the Sheriff within 28 days.

Correspondence (Section 34)

This makes provision for the Responsible Medical Officer to withhold patients' mail. However, patients may write unhindered to any of the following: the nearest relative, the Secretary of State, the Lord Advocate, any Member of Parliament, any Commissioner, the Mental Welfare Commissioner, any Sheriff or the hospital management.

Leave of absence (Section 35)

The arrangements here are similar to Section 17 in the England and Wales Act.

Absence without leave (AWOL) (Section 36)

This is similar to Section 18 in the England and Wales Act except that AWOL patients may not be taken into custody after the expiration of the following periods:
  (a) In the case of mental deficiency — 3 months.
  (b) In the case of an emergency detention — 7 days.
  (c) In any other case — 28 days.

Section 91

This makes provision for the protection of patients' property. A local health authority may petition for the appointment of a curator bonis to manage and administer the property of a person in their area who is incapable of doing so by reason of mental disorder.

Section 92

This makes provision for the hospital management to hold money and valuables on behalf of any detained patient where the RMO is of the opinion that he is incapable of administering his property and effects because of mental disorder.

Mental Health Amendment (Scotland) Bill 1982

(References: *Sections 1—35 Mental Health Amendment (Scotland) Bill*, HMSO (1982)

This Bill amends the 1960 Act as follows:

1 Substitutes Mental Handicap for mental deficiency.
2 Reduces length of emergency admission from 7 days to 72 hours.
3 Powers to allow a prescribed class nurse to hold an informal patient for 2 hours.
4 A 72 hour admission may be extended to 28 days on completion of a Report on the patient's condition.
5 Detention periods to read 6 months, then 1 year, then renewable yearly.
6 Introduces new provisions for consent to treatment (similar to 1983 Mental Health Act, England and Wales).
7 New curtailments on the existing powers to intercept patients' correspondence.
8 New safeguards for detained patients' rights, i.e. hospitals must give patients information on their rights, three yearly reviews by the Mental Welfare Commission of all detained patients, a new Code of Practice and more opportunities for appeals to the Sheriff.

4   Mental Health Bill (Eire) 1980

This Bill proposes new provisions for the care and treatment of the mentally disordered as follows:

Section 9

A district psychiatric centre is any hospital or unit designated for providing psychiatric care.

Section 13

This allows for voluntary admissions

Section 15

Applications for reception and detention require support from two medical recommendations.

Section 16

Removal to a Garda station of persons believed to be suffering from severe mental disorder for the purpose of making an application for reception (within 24 hours).

Section 21

Detention periods read as 28 days, 3 months and 12 months.

Section 27

This makes provisions for returning persons absent without leave.

Section 28

This makes provisions for granting authorised leave of absence.

Section 29

Transfer of detained persons to another psychiatric centre.

Section 32

Discharge by Medical Officer.

Section 33

This authorises Health Boards and medical officers to give information about detained persons. Persons refused such information may appeal to a Circuit Court Judge.

Section 35

Correspondence addressed to the Minister, President of the High Court, Health Boards or Review Boards must be forwarded unopened.

Section 36

All psychiatric centres shall be inspected yearly.

Section 37

Psychiatric Review Boards shall exist for each Health Board area with powers to discharge either conditionally or unconditionally. Membership to include a legal person, medical person and a non legal/medical member.

Section 40

Long-term detention shall be reviewed every two years. Persons examined by Review Boards are entitled to representation.

Section 44

This makes provisions for consent to certain therapeutic procedures.

Section 45

Reporting of alleged offences and other matters.

33
Chemotherapy

Drugs act by altering the chemical and physical environment of the brain cells, thus producing changes in the patient's mental state. In some cases the actual physical effects of the substance may be reinforced by the psychological benefits experienced by the patient. Indeed, it has been shown that patients given placebos (i.e. tablets containing inactive substances like glucose) also respond. Many patients expect tablets to be part of their treatment and some may refuse tablets because of psychiatric symptoms or as a gesture of independence or self-management.

Use of chemotherapy

It is accepted that most of the drugs used in treatment do not cure mental illness but are usually a part of the wider treatment which may include psychotherapy, rehabilitation, social help and so on. Some reasons for their use may include the following:
1 To reduce psychiatric symptoms such as delusions and hallucinations.
2 To raise the mood as in depression.
3 To calm the patient as in mania, schizophrenia and confusion.
4 To relieve agitation and anxiety and promote relaxation.
5 To stimulate interest, reduce inertia and confusion.

Advantages and disadvantages of chemotherapy

1 Advantages

Drug therapy, particularly tranquillisers, has brought important improvements to the management, treatment and nursing care of the psychiatric patient.

General improvements

1 More of the mentally ill are receiving treatment at home and hospital admissions have been reduced.
2 There has been growth in the resettlement of long-stay patients and a consolidation of community psychiatry.

Hospital improvements

1 The 'open door' policy has been enhanced and locked wards abolished.

2 The abolition of padded cells and other restraints has been facilitated.

3 The therapeutic community and nurse/patient relationships have been promoted.

4 There has been an added impetus to rehabilitation and a reduction in the hospital population.

5 There has been an added impetus to other treatments and management attitudes.

2 Disadvantages

1 Drugs are expensive and unpleasant side effects may occur.

2 They may be used as an expedient and some patients become dependent.

3 Some patients may stop taking the drug when they feel better and symptoms reoccur.

4 Accidental/intended overdosage is a risk, especially with the out-patient.

The main drug groups

Tranquillisers

These drugs produce a state of calm and sense of well being without clouding consciousness or inducing sleep. Major tranquillisers (such as phenothiazines) are used mainly for psychotic symptoms while the minor tranquillisers (e.g. benzodiazepines) benefit emotional symptoms such as anxiety.

Antidepressants

It is believed that these substances lift the mood by raising the level of amines (e.g., noradrenaline) in the brain. Tricyclic antidepressants, such as imipramine, raise the amine level by blocking its reabsorption, while the monoamine oxidase inhibitors, such as phenelzine, prevent the enzyme monoamine oxidase from destroying amines.

Anti-parkinsonism drugs

These reduce the parkinsonism side effects of major tranquillisers. Examples are orphenadrine, benzhexol and benztropine.

Anticonvulsants

These are used to treat convulsions. Examples are phenobarbitone and Phenytoin Sodium.

Hypnotics

There are many sleep-inducing drugs in use such as nitrazepam, barbiturates and chloral hydrates.

Minor Tranquillisers

Approved name	Trade name	Average daily dose	Effect	Side effect
Chlordiazepoxide	Librium	10 mg	Relieves anxiety and agitation	
Diazepam	Valium	10 mg	Prevents convulsions Muscle relaxant effects	Mild skin reactions in some patients

Commonly used major tranquillisers

Approved name	Trade name	Average daily dose	Effects	Side effects	Toxic effects	Administration
Chlorpromazine	Largactil	75 mg	Sedative effect, reduces confusion, reduces restlessness, aggression and delusional ideas	Drowsiness Hypotension Parkinsonism	Jaundice Photosensitivity Agranulocytosis	By tablets, syrup, injection or suppository
Trifluoperazine	Stelazine	10 mg	Less sedative effects than Largactil. Good for inert psychotics and is often used as maintenance therapy in chronic patients	Parkinsonism effects more common than with Largactil Drowsiness	—	By tablets, spansule, syrup or injection
Haloperidol	Serenace	2–15 mg	Good for controlling the excitement of mania and schizophrenia	Parkinsonism Dystonic reactions	—	By tablets, syrup or injection
Fluphenazine	Moditen and Modecate	Usually 25 mg every other week	Most useful in the re-habilitation of long stay schizophrenics Used widely in the community	Parkinsonism Restlessness	—	By i.m. injection — long-acting, slowly absorbed
Flupenthixol	Depixol					

NOTE: 1 Parkinsonism side effects can be reduced by giving Benzhexol, Orphenadrine or Benztropine.

2 Regular medication is important as these drugs do not cure.

3 Observation for, and prevention of, side effects is very important.

Commonly used antidepressants

Approved name	Trade name	Average Daily Dose	Effects	Side effects	Toxic effects	Administration
1 Tricyclic Group						
Imipramine	Tofranil	100 mg	Lifts depression particularly the psychotic type	Dry mouth, oedema, hypotension, constipation	—	Tablets or injection
Amitriptyline	Tryptizol	100 mg		Dry mouth, dizziness nausea, constipation		Tablets, syrup or injection
2 Monoamine Oxidase Inhibitors (MAOI'S)						
Phenelzine	Nardil	45 mg	Lifts depression, particularly neurotic type	Hypotension, nausea and oedema	Liver damage	Tablets
Isocarboxazid	Marplan	30 mg				

NOTE: 1 Education of patients on MAOI's is important. They should avoid cheese, oxo, Bovril and alcohol.
2 Patients on MAOI'S should have their blood pressure checked regularly.
3 Patients previous medication is considered before commencing MAOI drugs.
4 Tricyclic antidepressants may be used in combination with ECT.

Administration of medicines

For a more detailed account of the administration of medicine the nurse should refer to her aids for practical nursing or other suitable procedure manual. I will only mention here the special points in relation to psychiatric patients.

(1) Never leave the trolley or medicine cupboard unattended.
(2) Always ensure that the patient (especially if he is suicidal) has swallowed his medication.
(3) A lot of persuasion may be necessary to get some patients to take medication.
(4) Always be on the look-out for side effects.
(5) Medication should be checked by two nurses and there should be follow up monitoring of the patient in the community.

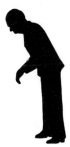

The nurse must observe and report side effects.
A common side effect from major tranquillisers
is Parkinsonism-type stiffness and rigidity

Fig. 33.1   Side effects can be modified

34
Physical Treatments

Drug therapy and psychological treatments have gradually replaced most physical treatments. However, in a minority of
patients their response to drugs may not be favourable in effecting
the required recovery. In those cases, physical methods may be
used either on their own or combined with drugs and other
therapies.

1 Electroconvulsive therapy (Electroplexy)

This method is used for treating severe depression (especially when
suicidal tendencies are present), and less frequently some schizo-
phrenias and mania. The use of anaesthetic, muscle relaxant and
electric shock are involved, therefore the patient is prepared as
follows:

Preparation of the patient

Before electroconvulsive therapy is administered, the patient and
relatives should be given explanations and reassurance about the
treatment. The patient will be told that it is a safe, painless
procedure carried out under anaesthesis. The treatment will aim to
relieve symptoms and promote a quick recovery. The patient may
be reassured by sharing his feelings with other persons undergoing
the same treatment and the nurse will add to this by her presence
before, during and after the procedure. Written consent must be
obtained for this treatment.

A physical examination is given; a six hour fast and an empty
bladder are necessary before treatment.

The nurse must remain with the patient and remove false teeth,
metal hair clips and administer pre-medication as prescribed by the
doctor.

The ECT procedure

The nurse should observe the patient prior to treatment, further
reassure him and check that his physical preparation is complete as
outlined above.

A quiet area of the ward should be screened from view or a
specially prepared clinic room may be used. The patient may lie on

his back on a bed or trolley and all tight clothing is loosened while the doctor, anaesthetist and other treatment personnel are introduced to the patient. Further reassurance takes place.

An intravenous injection is given to relax the muscle.

A mouth gag is inserted to prevent tongue biting and the saline soaked electrodes are now placed on the temples. The chin and jaw are supported. The shock is administered at 70–130 V for 0.25–2.0 s.

The patient convulses. On relaxation an airway is inserted and oxygen or air is given by a mask.

The patient begins to breathe again as the effects of the scoline wear off; he is turned on his left side and remains unconscious, with the airway in situation.

After-care

The nurse should:

(1) Nurse the patient in left lateral position and never leave him unattended. Observe and maintain a clear airway.

(2) Observe for cyanosis, distressed breathing and pulse irregularity.

(3) Have suction apparatus and oxygen available to cope with mucous obstruction of the airway or laboured breathing.

(4) On recovery, reassure the patient and offer him a cup of tea but continue to supervise him until his memory is fully recovered. Headache, memory loss and temporary confusion are common occurrences after the first few treatments.

Frequency of Treatments

Treatments are usually given twice a week. The total number of treatments is gauged by the patient's response and assessment review. 6–12 treatments are commonly used.

2 Psychosurgery

Surgery may be performed on the brain to sever nerve fibres between the frontal lobes and the thalamus. The operation is not without controversy but its advocates claim it is successful in freeing anxiety which is associated with severe tension. It may be used in selected cases to relieve agitation/anxiety/tension in chronic phobic anxiety states, agitated schizophrenia, obsessional states and chronic agitated depression.

The operation is usually only performed when all other treatments have failed to relieve symptoms. It is essential that the doctor discusses the operation with the patient and his relatives. The risks involved should be explained and a written request to perform psychosurgery should be obtained. Following the operation, intensive social and occupational rehabilitation will be necessary to prevent apathy.

3 Modified narcosis

In some acute psychiatric states the patient may require a period of mental and physical rest before treatment proper begins. Modified narcosis aims to keep the patient asleep approximately 15 hours out of the 24 hours each day. The treatment usually only lasts for two to three days and the technique involves the use of drugs. A combination of a sedative and a tranquilliser are given every four to six hours.

The patient is nursed in a quiet room under continuous observation. Foods and fluids must be encouraged and the nurse must ensure that the patient attends to his toilet, personal hygiene and appearance in the normal manner. Observation charts are maintained for the administration of drugs, duration of sleep, blood pressure, temperature, pulse, respiration and fluid balance. Routine change of position and frequent skin care is important to prevent pressure sores.

Complications

There are dangerous complications associated with this treatment which may include: bronchopneumonia, urinary retention, cardiovascular collapse, confusion and dehydration. If the blood pressure falls or the temperature rises, the treatment is-stopped.

35
Psychological Treatments

A 'word of mouth' approach is part of all aspects in the treatment, management and nursing care of the psychiatric patient. In previous chapters discussion has included the therapeutic community, nurse/patient relationships, remotivation and re-habilitative techniques and behavioural therapy. In this chapter we will discuss more specific areas of psychological treatment.

Psychotherapy

Psychotherapy, fundamentally, is based on the simple philos-ophy that a problem shared is a problem halved. From the nurse's own experience she may recall the relief experienced when she was able to talk over a problem with a willing listener. Almost immediately there is a sense of release at getting it 'off your chest' and somehow the problem is not as big as first thought.

Psychotherapy is an integral part of the doctor/nurse involve-ment in treatment. At a basic level it is used widely by both in their day-to-day contact with the patient. And, at a more involved level, it may be used in a direct way as a treatment technique. The benefit of this therapy rests with a 'here and now' effect whereby a fairly quick method is offered to help the patient understand and adjust to his immediate symptoms.

Practising psychotherapy

Establishing a relationship

The effectiveness of psychotherapy depends on the relationship between the therapist and patient. A good rapport is necessary and trust must be established.

Getting to know the patient is the first important step and the therapist must sit down and encourage the patient to talk about himself, his problems, and his symptoms. At this stage of the relationship the patient should be doing most of the talking with the therapist merely encouraging, listening and reassuring.

As the number of contacts increases, so, too, will the patient's trust in the therapist. Slowly he will be more forthcoming with his problems. His confidence in the therapist grows and this provides opportunities for her to become more positive with support and constructive suggestions which will offer help and relief.

Helping the patient

At the outset of treatment the therapist should have a clear and realistic view of what she can hope to achieve for the patient.

Having encouraged the patient to discuss his symptoms, it may be necessary to help him to accept that they may have an emotional basis. This may not be easy for him to accept and it is important that reassurance and explanation are forthcoming from the therapist. The patient will need reassuring that this does not mean his problem is unimportant or that emotional problems imply failure and weakness. Explanation of how emotional problems cause symptoms is necessary and, through reassurance and understanding, the patient's symptoms are reduced.

Terminating the relationship

As the patient's confidence grows, the support of the therapist will be gradually withdrawn. The patient is prepared for this in advance and the therapist should explain that the sessions are being reduced. Normally problems only arise if the termination is abrupt and unaccounted or if a close transference relationship has developed.

Group treatments

In past decades there was a tendency to treat the psychiatric patient as one of a crowd rather than one of a group. More recently the principle of a group approach to treatment has developed popularity in modern psychiatry. There are numerous types of group in use but they all have similar basic aims.

Aims of group treatment

(1) To create an environment conducive to re-educating unfavourable attitudes, behaviour patterns and orientation.
(2) To introduce the patient to situations where he can study others' behaviour, thereby gaining a greater understanding of himself.
(3) To introduce the patient to situations where his views, attitudes, opinions etc., are exposed to group comment.

(4) To introduce the patient to situations whereby he will realise he is not alone and that others have similar problems.

(5) To involve patients more directly in their own treatment and encourage participation in helping each other.

Some examples of group treatment

Groups play an important role in the therapeutic community; there are small and large groups, patient groups, staff groups and so on. The largest group of all, however, is the therapeutic community itself and, as was discussed in an earlier chapter, it includes the whole hospital or unit — staff and patients. For the purpose of this account we will look at various groups within the therapeutic unit or ward which will lead to consideration of group functioning and the nursing role.

Patient groups

1 **Ward meeting.** This is a large group meeting which takes place between all patients and staff either on a daily or weekly basis depending on the type of ward. The average attendance is about 25–40, (see Chapter 3).

2 **Small ward groups.** Patients may be divided into smaller groups (10–12 persons) for a variety of reasons. For example, to organise a recreational activity, discuss an agenda, or to promote interaction and communication. These groups may vary in organisation: e.g., they may elect a leader from their group or the group may be chaired by a doctor or nurse.

3 **Special groups.** Special groups are more intensive and are usually confined to members who have a common problem or interest which they can share. The best known example seen in most hospitals is the Alcoholic Group. Other examples may be phobic groups, adolescent groups, drug dependent groups, etc.. These groups are usually conducted by a therapist and meet on a daily basis.

4 **Crisis groups.** This type of group is more rarely seen but there are occasions when its formation may be helpful. Such groups may meet only on a one-off basis, and the aim is to prevent an explosion in group or ward harmony.

5 Nursing groups. Small groups of patients who present similar nursing problems may be grouped together for intensive remotivation, nursing care and rehabilitation. Two nurses usually work opposite shifts with each group, so that there is continuity in relationships and objectives. The nurse relates with her group throughout each day and reports on progress or problems to the weekly ward meeting. It is important for the two nursing leaders to be in accord with their approach and objectives, otherwise patients may not progress as hoped. Such groups may be used with success for patients with problems such as untidiness, bad habits, withdrawal, foul language and so on.

Staff groups

These have already been discussed under therapeutic organisation in a previous chapter. It is important that good communications and understanding should be promoted between staff who are involved in group activity. Group leaders should meet together and discuss their roles, exchange ideas, discuss group problems and so on.

Group dynamics

The term group dynamics was introduced by Kurt Lewin in 1939. It is a loose term used to describe group behaviour, tensions, cohesions and so on.

Arranging group therapy sessions

Patients are selected in consultation with doctor and ward sister. The meeting times are arranged and the group format and programme is decided. A quiet room is selected and seating arranged in a circular fashion, to allow eye contact, with the group leader as part of the circle. All members should be encouraged to participate in the group activity.

The nurse's role in group therapy

1 Preparation of the patient. Patients who are joining the group for the first time are often apprehensive as to what it is all about. Some may fear the face-to-face confrontations and be anxious about their contribution and role in the treatment. Others may scorn the group and consider it is of no use to them or they may have preconceived ideas about baring their soul in front of strangers and so on.

The nurse can do much to prepare the patient by explaining the treatment to him. He should be introduced to other group members and made aware of his commitment to the group (i.e. how often it meets, the amount of time involved etc.). He should be shown the room where meetings will take place and, if a programme of group activities is involved, he should be provided with a copy. The objectives of the group may be explained to him.

2 Conducting a session. Should the nurse be involved in conducting a session, she should allow the patients to develop their own themes. She should neither push the processes nor be dragged along by them, rather she should be passive but mediatory in her role.

To commence, the nurse should introduce herself. When patients are resisting personal participation or involvement by irrelevant mutterings, she could comment on this. Again, should a patient remain silent or be unable to articulate with outspoken members, he should be supported by the nurse.

3 After-care. Following the session some patients may feel self-recrimination about a personal revelation to the group; they may have said something which they instantly regretted and be greatly bothered by this. Patients who appear to be upset by the group dynamism may require reassurance, support and observation following the session.

Note on group therapy

Group therapy may be a traumatic experience for some patients and involve much contemplation and exposure of personal weaknesses and intimate problems. It may also be an anxious experience for a nurse learner; therefore, it is important that the group therapist should be an experienced person. In closed group therapy, nurse learners, if they are permitted to observe, should only do so in a learning capacity under the supervision of an experienced nurse. It is important for the supervisor to impress upon the learner the confidential nature of the patient's revelations during a group session.

Abreaction

This procedure may be used for either treatment or diagnostic purposes. Patients may resist, or be unable to recall, conflicts or events which were emotionally disturbing but which are associated with the development of their present symptoms. To relive a period of great unhappiness may be difficult, therefore, drugs may be given to remove inhibitions and make recall and expression easier. When drugs are used (narcoanalysis) the one preferred is usually intravenous amylobarbitone but Evipan or thiopentone can also be used.

Procedure

(1) The doctor explains the treatment and obtains consent. The nurse should reassure the patient as necessary.
(2) A quiet room is prepared (the patient usually lies on the bed or sits in a comfortable chair). A tape recorder or cassette may be used.
(3) An injection tray is made ready with the drug to be used (and the antidote) plus the patient's case notes.
(4) The nurse should protect the doctor from interruptions during the procedure.
   Abreactions may be used for neurotic conditions, particularly hysteria.

Psychoanalysis

This approach is also known as couch therapy or the science of the unconscious functions of the mind and personality. In psychoanalysis the aim is to uncover unconscious motivation and repressed memories thus leading to a knowledge of unconscious feelings, impulses, fantasies and ideas.

   The treatment is conducted with the patient lying on a couch and free-associating (i.e. the patient talks about the first thing that comes into his head regardless of any apparent connection it may have with his present illness). Each interview lasts about 45 minutes and the analyst may also take a suggestive role. A course of treatment by psychoanalysis may last from one to five years.

Hypnosis

Hypnosis is a form of suggestion which may be used to treat hysterical symptoms (such as paralysis) and other neurotic conditions. During hypnosis the doctor causes the patient to pass into a suggestive state (akin to sleep except that the patient remains aware of the doctor's voice) and may give instructions to the patient as he thinks necessary, e.g. to use an hysterical paralysed limb again or stop a tic or other faulty habit. A quiet room (preferably soundproof) is necessary and the nurse should protect the doctor from interruptions during the procedure.

Psychodrama

This is a form of group therapy involving role-playing to act out a particular problem. The patient concerned plays out events from his own life and the other patients play the part of persons in his life and work (e.g. boss, wife, friends and so on). No script is written and the actors ad lib as they go along. (see also p. 22).

Relaxation therapy

Relaxation therapy is being increasingly used to help patients with tension, anxiety and agitation. It may take many forms to include meditation, exercises, body control and music. It is generally carried out with a group of patients and a quiet room free from interruptions is necessary.

Behaviour therapy

The term 'behaviour therapy' refers to several methods of treatment all based on psychological theories of learning derived essentially from Pavlov's work on conditioning. As we have related behaviour techniques to treatment and nursing care in other chapters, they will only be briefly reviewed before discussing other aspects of this treatment (see Chapter 15).

1 Aversion therapy

This is the earliest known behavioural treatment and is used to treat alcoholism (see also Chapter 22). The technique involves the administration of alcohol with emetics (e.g. apomorphine) to produce nausea and vomiting. The learning principle in this approach involves punishment for an established behaviour (drinking), thereby inducing conflict between the desire to drink and the fear of unpleasant effects. It is hoped that the aversion treatment will suppress the undesirable behaviour and hence prevent the patient from drinking alcohol. It has become evident however that the effects tend to be temporary and repetition of the treatment is often required at subsequent intervals.

More recently the techniques of aversion conditioning have

been applied to the treatment of sexual deviation and other deviant behaviours.

2 Reciprocal inhibition and desensitisation

This approach was introduced by Wolpe and differs from aversion conditioning in that deliberate attempts are made to extinguish fear and anxiety through desensitisation to the source of fear. Desensitisation is used for anxiety generating situations and aims to help the patient to relax while he is exposed to the situation which would normally provoke anxiety. Sometimes drugs (methohexitone) may be used. An example for a desensitisation programme to treat a swimming phobia is included in Chapter 15.

Nurse therapists have treated phobias (social phobias), obsessional states, hysterical reactions, sex problems and habit disorders such as stammering and enuresis.

More recently, nurse therapists have been extending their role to some of the intractable problems of long-term and mentally handicapped conditions.

Crisis intervention

Crisis intervention is an aspect of primary preventive psychiatry which acts to help families or individuals through crisis periods of stress with a view to lessening the risk of psychiatric breakdown. For example, it is known that recently bereaved widows are vulnerable to depressive breakdown; therefore, if some planned intervention can be developed for this type of crisis, the incidence of bereavement depression may be reduced.

Crisis intervention may involve the whole family unit during periods of stress which create tensions and disturb the family harmony. The intervention programme will aim to restore the family equilibrium through discussion, adjustment, support and change.

36

Situational Dilemmas
and Emergencies

Difficult nursing situations arise on psychiatric wards for which there may be no guidelines or a right or wrong method for resolution. Included are:

1 Continuous observation

Care programmes may make it necessary to confine a patient to the ward during acute phases of his illness such as manic or schizophrenic episodes, the emergence of suicidal tendencies, and confused periods. The patient is closely supervised within the ward and may only leave when accompanied by a nurse. This is considered necessary to prevent the patient from coming to harm.

However, problems arise if the patient lacks insight or refuses to co-operate. During disturbed phases he may run from the ward and the nurse may be forever in pursuit and distress. To facilitate supervision, the nurse may be tempted to lock the door but this will conflict with the therapeutic atmosphere and impede the movement and freedom of other ward patients. The dilemma arises in that by acting in the interests of one patient the nurse may be in conflict with therapeutic principles and the interests of the remaining ward residents.

In Chapter 31 it is mentioned that there is nothing in the Mental Health Act which authorises the detention of an informal patient in a locked ward. However, the 1978 Review of the Act suggests that action to prevent such patients from wandering and coming to harm is unlikely to be challenged.

When a problem such as this does arise, the caring team should endeavour to allocate sufficient resources to enable the patient to be managed in the freedom of the open ward. On occasions when resources are scarce, during staff shortages for example, the team should review the situation and prepare an alternative programme which, insofar as is possible, will exclude locking the main ward entrances and exits. Should management impede the freedom of the other ward patients, this must be discussed with them and a staff member should always be available to open and close doors. In the final analysis, if an irresponsible patient wanders and comes to harm the hospital may be open to a claim for failing to provide care and protection. It is against this background that a holding power is included for nurses in the 1983 Mental Health Act.

2 Confined treatment

The traditional type of seclusion is no longer used in psychiatric treatment. However, in an emergency, staff may have to confine a patient (either formal or informal) to his bedroom for a short period or impose some form of treatment, such as a sedative, for the safety of all concerned. The 1978 Review of the English Mental Health Act mentions that in such cases staff are justified in law to do this to an informal patient only if it is immediately necessary to save life, or prevent violence or serious deterioration in the patient's condition. Staff may also (under Section 3(1) of the Criminal Law Act, 1967) use such force as is reasonable in the circumstances prevailing at the time to prevent a violent or dangerous act which would amount to a crime. In situations other than these, the 1978 Review states that where it is essential to seclude or impose treatment, the necessary authority under an appropriate section of the Mental Health Act should be sought. This also applies where it can be foreseen that emergencies are likely to recur. It should be noted that the taking of compulsory powers also brings safeguards (application to a Mental Health Review Tribunal, etc.), not available to an informal patient.

Each problem is an individual one and frequent ward discussion will promote guidance and understanding to ensure the right decision is made for the patient. The management emphasis should be to reduce the need for confinement. However, in crisis situations the reason for confinement should be clearly recorded in the patient's records and reviewed frequently. Confinement should not be prolonged one moment longer than is necessary.

3 Searching patients

It may be necessary for a nurse to search a patient as part of her duty. For example, suicidal or drug dependent patients may conceal drugs, violent patients may conceal offensive weapons and so on. If a nurse suspects a patient to be concealing something which is a danger to himself or others, she should relate with the nursing team on duty before following any course of action. Facts should be established before searching is authorised as this procedure would be undignified and upsetting to an innocent patient.

The 1978 Review of the Mental Health Act concludes that staff have authority in common law and by virtue of Section 3(1) of the Criminal Law Act (1967) to take reasonable measures to prevent a patient from keeping in his possession articles of potential danger (e.g., matches, weapons, alcohol, tools or explosives. This opinion is also set out in circular (HC (76)11). However, there is no legal justification for routine searching of patients' belongings where there are no good grounds for believing that there is a risk of violence, drug concealment, etc.

Tact and understanding are necessary and the patient should be reassured and given the opportunity to save face, with actual searching only taking place as a last resort. The search should be conducted by a senior nurse and in the patient's presence. The reasons for carrying out the search and the results of the procedure must be recorded in the patient's notes. Informal patients who persistently abuse treatment may be offered their discharge.

4 Extra-marital affairs

Extra-marital affairs may take place between patients (particularly on mixed sex wards) during hospitalisation. The nurse has a clear role with compulsorily detained patients, but it is difficult for the medical and nursing staff to prevent informal patients having affairs if they are determined to do so. However, if a male patient is taking advantage of a female patient (or vice versa) during the acute phase of her illness, some involvement by nursing staff is necessary to protect the patient and reassure her spouse. Discussion between the ward team members will decide what action should be taken and in some situations the patient may be transferred to an all female ward. Sometimes spouses of patients may complain during visiting time and show concern about their 'other half' being nursed on the same ward as male patients. Jealous husbands and boyfriends can be difficult to reassure but the ward team should endeavour to do what they think is in the best interest of both patient and spouse.

5 Thefts

Some psychiatric patients may steal from other patients during acute illness, confusion and absent-mindedness. Also, some patients may wrongly accuse both staff and patients of theft during paranoid phases in their illness.

The nursing team should ensure that all patients understand the implications of retaining large sums of money or valuable possessions in their locker or on their person. Hospital recommendations regarding money and valuables should be implemented and patients should be reminded about leaving possessions in exposed areas (e.g. on beds and locker tops). In situations where patients complain about loss or theft of articles, the nurse should endeavour to establish whether the articles were brought into hospital in the first instance. Patients may misplace articles and a helpful nurse can assist the patient to retrace his movements and locate the possession. In some instances the nurse may have to consider whether the patient's complaint or accusation is part of a delusions system.

6 Drunkenness

Patients may return to the ward from a social evening or outing under the influence of alcohol. In most instances the patient may be co-operative but occasionally he may be argumentative, abusive and threatening. The helpful nurse can be reassuring and a hot drink of strong coffee followed by bed and observation may help the patient to 'sleep it off'.

In difficult situations the help of other nursing staff should be sought and the medical officer informed. It is important for the nurse to consider the patient's treatment and if this includes medication which may potentiate or conflict with alcohol (e.g. monoamine oxidase antidepressants, barbiturates, or disulfiram), the medical officer should be informed. Also, in cases where the patient appears to be deeply intoxicated, the treatment team should observe for symptoms of alcoholic poisoning and guard against sickness and vomiting which may cause choking. Following the incident it should be made clear to the patient that he failed to adhere to his contract with the treatment team not to drink.

7 Unplanned admissions

Persons may present themselves to admission wards and request, or in some instances, demand, admission to hospital without a referral from a doctor. In some situations the person may be drunk or down on his luck and merely seeking a bed for the night, but in other situations, he may be an ex-patient with recurring symptoms or problems. Hospital rules vary for these situations and it is important for the nurse to avoid implementing admission procedure until she relates with a senior nurse and seeks medical advice. Meanwhile the person should be asked to wait and be reassured until a decision is taken. It may be necessary to contact the patient's family or arrange transport to a place of safety if admission is prohibited.

The 1978 Review of the Mental Health Act mentions that some hospitals bar informal admissions after 5 pm with the result that any admission after this time has to be compulsory. The Review concludes that such rules should be discontinued and that hospitals should make arrangements for both formal and informal emergency admissions.

8 Assault and threats

The nature of some psychiatric illnesses may cause a patient to assault another patient or member of staff. In such cases the nursing team should resolve the situation as outlined for the aggressive patient in Chapter 20. It is important for the nurse to note, however, that in cases involving informal patients a court action for assault may be taken by the injured party against the offender, and the nursing staff who observed the incident may be involved as witnesses. Any injuries involving either party during an assault should receive the appropriate medical and nursing attention and an accident form should be completed. Unfortunately, there are occasions when the assaulted patient may receive serious injuries from which death may follow. In that event, the observing nursing staff may be witnesses in a Coroner's Court, while the offending patient may be charged with either murder or manslaughter.

Occasionally a patient may repeatedly threaten another patient and cause him to become anxious and frightened. Nursing staff should be aware when such a situation develops and be positive in reassuring the 'frightened' patient and in helping him to feel more at ease. A nursing presence should be maintained at all times and a team meeting may be necessary to discuss the management of the 'bullying' patient.

9 Absconding

Elderly confused and acutely disturbed patients who are under nursing supervision may run or wander from the ward or hospital grounds on to a roadway or other public place. When this occurs the nurse should follow the patient and persuade him to return to the ward. However, there may be occasions when the patient may refuse and struggle with the nurse if she attempts to impede his efforts to run. This can be a delicate situation to handle as members of the public may misunderstand the nursing image if they observe nurses in uniform struggling with someone in public.

In delicate situations such as this, the nurse should be motivated by the patient's illness and her own personal safety. If the patient is likely to come to harm, the nurse should do all she can to ensure his safe return to hospital. However, if the patient is in no immediate danger and a difficult and unpleasant struggle is likely in any attempt to return him to hospital, it may be advisable for the nurse to allow him to proceed and return to her ward for discussion with the ward team.

10 Complaints

Patients may complain about a variety of things and on many occasions. The most appropriate place to encourage complaints is during the ward meeting and the ward team should consider all complaints from patients. Some grievances may be a manifestation of the patient's illness or based on some misunderstanding, rumour or lack of information. All patients (and their relatives) should be made aware of procedures for formal complaint if they feel that their problems are not being resolved at ward level.

In most situations where patients or relatives have a complaint which is not receiving attention, they may write to the consultant in charge of treatment, the Senior Nursing Officer, the Hospital Administrator or the Hospital Management Board. If they should continue to be dissatisfied at this level, they may also complain to Community Health Councils, ex-patient associations, local councillors, members of Parliament, the Parliamentary Commissioner, the Health Service Commission or the European Commissioner for Human Rights.

11 Damaged property

Some patients may damage hospital property (e.g. by smashing windows or glass panel doors) during an acute episode of their illness. Disturbances of this nature can have an unpleasant effect on the ward environment, therefore, the nurse must put emphasis on coping with the situation and restoring the ward to normal functioning as follows:

(1) By giving immediate attention to the offending patient by removing him from danger and giving appropriate reassurance and treatment.

(2) By protecting the remaining patients from discomfort or danger and giving reassurance.

(3) By notifying the appropriate maintenance department to repair damage to property.

(4) By discussing the incident at a team meeting and completing an incident report and an accident form.

12 Suicidal incidents

Emergency nursing action is called for when a patient makes an attempt on his life. The nurse should use whatever force is necessary to restrain the patient for the purpose of removing the inflicting hazard. The nurses' preventive actions are expected under common law and the medical/nursing intervention is discussed in chapters 18 and 19.

Suicide incident evaluation

To learn and develop preventive techniques, the ward team should evaluate each suicidal incident:

- Does the patient have a history of suicide attempts?
- What is his present diagnosis and treatment?
- Did he experience any loss prior to admission?
- Is there a family history of suicide or previous destructive tendencies?
- How did he behave in the days/hours prior to the incident?
- Was he under close observation prior to the incident?
- How did he attempt suicide or gain access to the hazard?
- What time of the day/night did the incident occur?
- How was the incident managed?
- What was the time interval between incident and commencement of emergency treatment?
- Where did the incident take place and what was the staff/patient ratio?
- What are the patient's views and feelings about the incident?

Physical emergencies

Sudden collapse

Sudden collapse most commonly occurs in coronary thrombosis. However, other causes may include: hypoglycaemia, perforated peptic ulcer, internal bleeding, pulmonary embolism, obstructed airway, drug overdosage or poisoning, epilepsy, apoplexy, hysteria, fainting or alcohol intoxication.

Immediate care

The nurse should remain calm, go to the patient's aid and get help quickly by calling out. She should check breathing and any obstruction to the airway from food or mucus must be removed quickly. It is sometimes possible to reach the epiglottis with the finger to dislodge matter obstructing the opening to the larynx. Alternatively, the neck should be extended and the chin held forward. An emergency tray and oxygen should be made available and the doctor's instructions followed when he arrives. Management from this point will depend on the condition and the following situations will be discussed briefly:

1 Cardiac arrest

The patient will be unconscious with pupils dilated and respiratory distress. No pulse is felt at the carotid artery and no heart sounds are present. The nurse should act quickly to summon medical aid.

Action. The nurse should not wait for help to arrive – proceed from clear airway. She should give the chest over the sternum one blow with the closed fist. If this fails to start the heart she should proceed as follows: place the patient on his back on a hard surface; elevate the legs and check again that the airway is clear; commence external cardiac massage. Mouth-to-mouth resuscitation may also be necessary. A Brook airway may be used. She should continue with this management until the doctor arrives or the heart and breathing commence again.

Medical treatment. Intubation, ventilation and electrocardiogram (ECG) recording. Intravenous infusion of strong sodium bicarbonate 8.4 % may be given to prevent acidosis. Defibrillation with pads and electric shock. Suitably diluted intravenous dopamine (Intropin) or dobutamine (Dobutrex) to raise blood pressure.

2 Drug overdosage

If the patient is conscious the nurse should ask him which drug he took and how many. She should save the empty container. She must keep the patient awake and give an emetic, such as salt and water, or encourage vomiting by tickling the back of the throat with her finger. Vomit should be saved for analysis. Finally, the nurse should obtain medical aid and arrange casualty admission.

Barbiturate poisoning. Gastric lavage and intubation are often required. Intravenous fluids and catheterisation may be necessary. Occasionally dialysis is required.

Aspirin poisoning. Gastric lavage and ventilation are necessary. Forced alkaline diuresis may be necessary using normal saline and sodium bicarbonate 1.4%. Necessary records are: a level of consciousness chart, intake and output recording, and TPR, B/P and urine pH (acidity).

Benzodiazepine poisoning. Overdosage with one of the benzodiazepines (e.g. nitrazepam) is less dangerous than an overdose of aspirin or barbiturates. Death from respiratory depression is less common but can occur in patients with poor ventilatory function (such as bronchitis or emphysema).

Tricyclic antidepressant poisoning. The patient will require casualty admission and stomach wash-out. Blood pressure should be monitored in case of hypotension. ECG should be monitored in case of cardiac arrhythmias. A level of consciousness chart should be maintained and observation for respiratory depression and retention of urine. Should convulsions occur, diazepam 15 mg may be given intravenously and phenobarbitone intramuscularly.

3 Insulin coma

If the patient is conscious give a sweetened drink or a lump of sugar. If the patient improves it will indicate excess insulin. If diabetic coma is diagnosed the doctor will prescribe repeated injections of soluble insulin until the blood sugar falls and the patient regains consciousness. Collapse due to insulin coma is sudden while sugar coma develops gradually.

Observations in the unconscious patient

The following observations are helpful:
Skin. Pink colour denotes oxygenation. Observe for cyanosis. Moist sweaty skin suggests shock and vasoconstriction.
Breath. In a diabetic coma there is acetone smell. Note whether there is an alcohol smell.

Pulse. Increased pulse in haemorrhage and shock. Irregular pulse in heart disease and slow pulse in perforated ulcers.

Breathing. There is a deep sighing breathing in haemorrhage and diabetic coma. Shallow breathing in pneumonia and expiratory wheezing in asthma. Cheyne-Stokes breathing in heart disease.

Blood Pressure. A falling pressure denotes shock or bleeding.

Pupils. Observe reaction to light and whether pupils are equal, pinpoint or dilated.

Paralysis. Hemiplegia in apoplexy.

Vomit. Coffee grounds from stomach bleeding and bile stained in intestinal obstruction.

Urine. Reduced output in shock, uremia and dehydration. Sugar and acetone in diabetes. Haematuria in ruptured kidney.

Pain. Chest pain in coronary thrombosis. Abdominal pain and rigidity in perforated peptic ulcers.

Level of consciousness. Note depth. For example, if drowsy, the patient will respond to the spoken word. If rousable, he will only respond by moving arms or legs in response to painful stimuli. When not rousable there is no response to painful stimuli. This denotes deep unconsciousness.

Care of the unconscious patient

Following the initial first aid and emergency treatment the patient may remain unconscious for hours or weeks. Continuous nursing care and observation will be necessary as follows:

(1) Nurse the patient on his side to maintain a clear airway.

(2) Have oxygen and suction apparatus and a tray for the unconscious patient (i.e. airway, vomit bowl, mouth gag, torch) nearby.

(3) Prevent pressure sores by turning from side to side every two hours.

(4) Attention to regular oral hygiene.

(5) Nasogastric feeding.

(6) Record the following: TPR, intake and output, level of consciousness, bowel movement and vomit.

(7) Bed bathing and general attention to personal hygiene as appropriate.

Sudden vomiting and diarrhoea

Patients who develop sudden vomiting with abdominal pain and headache followed by diarrhoea may be suffering from food poisoning. The poisoning usually follows the ingestion of food contaminated with either salmonella or staphylococci bacteria and it may affect all the patients who ate the offensive food. If the vomiting occurs up to 12 hours after the meal it is probably a staphyloccal infection. Salmonella poisoning has a more delayed reaction with symptons occuring from 12–48 hours after infection.

Management and treatment

(1) Reassure the patient. Implement barrier nursing programme.
(2) Withhold solid foods and send specimens of vomit and faeces to the laboratory.
(3) Give fluids by mouth as much as possible as dehydration is a risk.
(4) Record TPR and intake and output.
(5) Antibiotics in some cases to control diarrhoea.
(6) Kaolin mixture in some cases to control diarrhoea.
(7) I.V. fluids in cases of severe dehydration.
(8) Give full nursing care and attention.
(9) Wash hands thoroughly and prevent the infected patient from handling food which others may consume.

37
Discussion Topics on Nursing Care

How might you distinguish between the following:
 (1) Reactive and endogenous depression?
 (2) Epileptic and hysterical seizures?
 (3) Formal care (compulsory) and informal care?
 (4) Anxiety neurosis and obsessional compulsive neurosis?
 (5) Hysterical symptoms and disseminated sclerosis?
 (6) Physical illness and physical complaints in neurotic conditions?
 (7) Electroconvulsive therapy and modified insulin therapy?
 (8) Catatonic stupor and depressive retardation?
 (9) Paranoid schizophrenia and paranoid delusions as a symptom of other illnesses?
(10) Schizophrenic excitement and manic excitement?
(11) Institutional neurosis and chronic schizophrenia?
(12) Hallucinations and illusions?
(13) Delusions of persecution and ideas of reference?
(14) Mania and thyrotoxicosis?
(15) Soft drug dependence and hard drug dependence?
(16) Puerperal psychosis and involutional melancholia?
(17) Hypomania and general paralysis of the insane?
(18) Psychopathic personality and epileptic personality?
(19) Hysteria and malingering?
(20) Pre-psychotic personality of schizophrenia and manic-depressive psychosis?
(21) Pre-senile and senile dementia?
(22) Childhood autism and phenylketonuria?
(23) Multidisciplinary meetings and staff/patient meetings?
(24) Aversion therapy and abreaction?
(25) Psychotherapy and psychoanalysis?
(26) Pavlovian conditioning and operant conditioning?
(27) Tricyclic antidepressants and monoamine oxidase inhibitors?
(28) Extra-pyramidal reactions and Parkinson's disease?
(29) Mental Health Review Tribunals and Courts of Protection?
(30) Day hospitals and day centres?

Nursing situations

How should the nursing team manage the following situations?
  (1) A disturbed patient who keeps running from the ward.
  (2) An informal patient who seeks discharge against medical advice.
  (3) A patient who violently attacks another patient.
  (4) A patient who cuts his wrists.
  (5) A patient who collapses with cardiac arrest.
  (6) A patient who develops delirium tremens.
  (7) A patient with catatonic stupor.
  (8) A patient suspected of concealing addictive drugs on his person.
  (9) A patient who persistently refuses to eat.
  (10) A patient who returns to the ward in a drunk and disorderly manner.
  (11) A patient who develops an acute panic attack.
  (12) A patient who complains that his letters are being opened.
  (13) A detained patient who goes absent without leave.

Glossary

This is intended to provide an explanation as well as a definition of some of the terms described in the text.

Psychiatry

Abortion, Therapeutic: a surgical termination of pregnancy for medical reasons. The pregnancy is interrupted before the twenty eighth week.

Abreaction: the living-out of an unconscious impulse using techniques which include hypnosis and injections of barbiturates.

Accommodation: the adjustment of the eye to various distances.

ACTH: Adrenocorticotrophic hormone secreted by the anterior pituitary gland.

Acting-out: the discharge of tension and release of feelings during psychotherapy.

Adler, Alfred (1870–1937): psychiatrist who founded the school of individual psychology.

Affect: a class name for feeling, emotion or mood.

Agoraphobia: the dread of open spaces.

Akinesia: an absence of voluntary movement.

Alcoholics Anonymous (AA): an organisation formed in 1935 to rehabilitate alcoholics.

Allport, Gordon (1897–1967): American psychologist and educator.

Altruism: a concern for the needs of others.

Altruistic Suicide: suicide committed to avoid becoming a burden on others (Durkheim).

Ambivalence: the existence of contradictory feelings at the same time. A term coined by Blueler. For example, 'I want to eat' and 'I don't want to eat'; 'I hear voices' and 'I don't hear voices.'

Analytical Psychology: Jung's system of psychology which, unlike that of Freud, regards the mind as something much more than a bank of past experiences.

Aphasia: language disturbance due to brain disorder.

Aphrodisiac: an agent that stimulates sexual feelings.

Association, Free: the removal of censorship on logical thinking so that a person may express spontaneously his thoughts as they pass through his mind.

Ataxia: the impairment or loss of muscular co-ordination.

Auto-immunity: the reacting of antibodies with the organism's own tissues. There is a common belief that autoantibody attacks tissues causing auto-immune diseases (AID) e.g. Hashimoto's disease, rheumatoid arthritis, ulcerative colitis, lupus erythematosus.

Automatism: the carrying out of activities without conscious knowledge.

Auto-suggestion: self-suggestion.

Aversion Therapy: negative conditioning using painful or unpleasant stimuli until the undesirable behaviour is suppressed (e.g. unwanted behaviour such as alcoholism).

Babinski's Reflex: extending the toes instead of flexing them when the sole of the foot is stroked.

Behaviour Therapy: based on the learning theories of Skinner and Thorndike. The underlying theory is that neurotic behaviour is learned behaviour, and therefore is amenable to unlearning. Behaviour therapy is aimed at the extinction of the faulty behaviour. Among the leading exponents of behaviour therapy and theory are Eynsenck and Wolpe.

Belle Indifférence: indifference and lack of concern.

Bleuler, Eugene (1857–1939): Swiss psychiatrist who suggested the term 'schizophrenia' to replace dementia praecox.

Catatonia: the abnormal maintenance of postures or physical attitudes producing a wax-like appearance.

Charcot, Jean-Martin (1825–1893): French neurologist and psychiatrist (Charcot's joints).

Cholinergic: nerves which release acetylcholine at their terminals.

Circumstantiality: when too many associated ideas come to consciousness so that the patient takes a long time to get to the point.

Clouding of Consciousness: impairment of orientation, perception and attention.

Complex: unacknowledged repressed ideas which continue to influence behaviour and thought.

Concussion: paralysis of brain function due to a blow on the head.

Conditioning: Pavlovian or classical conditioning as seen in the experimental procedure in which a reflex may be modified so that it is evoked by a stimulus different from the natural one. For example, food is presented to an experimental animal to cause salivation and a bell is rung at the same time—the conditioned response is salivation in response to the bell ringing when food is not present.

Conditioning, Operant: 'Consequence-governed behaviour' is the term B. F. Skinner used for the process of reinforcing a person's spontaneous behaviour. The behaviour is reinforced by a reward.

Confabulation: the act of replacing memory loss by fantasy.

Conflict: a mental struggle resulting from a clash between opposing drives or wishes acting simultaneously. The conflict gives rise to emotional tension and anxiety.

Conolly, John (1794–1866): British psychiatrist (Medical Superintendent, Middlesex Asylum, 1839–50) who was foremost in implementing lectures for mental nurses. He was a pioneer in abolishing mechanical restraint of patients. He improved living conditions and tried to set up an educational system for patient rehabilitation.

Cyclothymia: mood fluctuations.

Death Instinct: Freudian destructive drives, striving for complete and eternal rest.

Déjà Vu: already seen, feeling of familiarity.

Depersonalisation: when a person feels that he has lost his individual identity.

Derealisation: feelings of changed reality.

Dipsomania: bout-drinking in alcoholism.

Dream: a psychic phenomenon occurring during sleep in which thoughts and emotions present themselves as if they were real.

Dymphna, St: the patron saint of the mentally disordered. Murdered by her insane father in Gheel, Belgium.

Dyskinesia: involuntary muscular movements such as tics, spasms, and myoclonus.

Dyslexia: difficulty reading or understanding what is read.

Dystonia: acute spasmodic movements of the limbs, torticollis, tongue protrusion and oculogyric crisis. A side effect of tranquillisers.

Echopraxia: the repetition of another's movements.

Effort Syndrome: a type of anxiety state.

Ego: the conscious part of the mind (psychoanalytic psychology). The part of the mind which mediates between the person and reality.

Euthanasia: the means of bringing about an early painless death.

Extra-pyramidal System: nerve tracts concerned with autonomic movements involved in postural adjustments. Extra-pyramidal dysfunction is seen in Parkinsonism, chorea, etc.

Folie à Deux: communicated mental disorder.

Freud, Sigmund (1856—1939): Austrian psychiatrist; founder of psychoanalysis. Originator of concepts such as libido, regression, transference, sublimation, Ego, Id, super-ego and Oedipus complex.

Fugue: wandering on a journey with loss of memory.

Ganser, Sigbert Joseph (1853—1931): German psychiatrist who invented the Ganser syndrome of approximate answers.

Gerontology: the study of old age.

Habit Training: the encouragement of patients' habits related to eating, elimination, dressing, washing and sleep. It is related to the care of deteriorated or incontinent patients, children and the mentally handicapped.

Heterosexuality: sexual attraction for the opposite sex.

Hydrocephalus: an increase in cerebrospinal fluid within the skull.

Hydrotherapy: the treatment of disease by water.

Idiopathic: undetermined cause.

Introvert: a quiet, shy, inward looking and unsociable person.

Jackson, John Hughlings (1834—1911): British neurologist.

Jung, Carl (1875—1961): Swiss psychiatrist who founded his own analytical school.

Kallmann, Franz (1897—1965): German geneticist who made studies on schizophrenia and manic-depressive psychosis.

Kernig, V. M. (1840—1917): Russian physician. Kernig's sign in meningitis is where an extention of the leg and knee produces pain and resistance

Kleptomania: a morbid impulse to steal.

Kraeplin, Emil (1856—1926): German psychiatrist who differentiated between manic-depressive psychosis and dementia praecox (schizophrenia).

Lange, Carl (1834—1900): Danish pathologist who invented Lange's gold curve test for syphilis.

Libido: The energy of the sexual drive.

LSD (lysergic acid diothylamide): An hallucinogenic drug, used in abreaction. LSD trips and psychosis are features.

Mania à Potu: an attack of excitement from alcohol or madness.

Melancholia: morbid mental state characterised by depression.

Meyer, Adolf (1866—1950): American psychiatrist — individualised mental illness.

Milieu Therapy: environment or social setting which is therapeutic and takes account of the patient's emotions.

Moniz, Ega (1874—1955): Portuguese neurologist who developed the leucotomy.

Monoamine oxidase: an enzyme discovered by Hare in 1928. Inhibition of this enzyme produces psychic energy.

Narcissism: self-love.

Narcoanalysis: pentothal interview; truth drug; injection of pentothal is given intravenously and this produces relaxation and desire to communicate. Previously repressed memories and conflict are expressed to the therapist during interview.

Neurasthenia: nervous debility and fatigue.

Nymphomania: insatiable sex drive in women.

Phobia: morbid fear associated with morbid anxiety.

Placebo: dummy treatment.

Porphyria: a metabolic disorder which results in the production of abnormal porphyrins which appear in the urine. There is no known treatment and 50 per cent of cases are fatal.

Psychosurgery: a general term now used to describe any brain surgery done to relieve mental illness.

Sakel, Manfred (1900–1957): Polish psychiatrist who introduced insulin treatment of schizophrenia.

Sexual Disorders

Bestiality: performing of the sexual act with animals.

Exhibitionism: indecent exposure of the genitals to obtain sexual excitement.

Fetishism: obtaining of sexual pleasure or excitement from objects of the opposite sex, e.g. hair, handbags, undergarments, stockings. Some fetishists may steal underwear from clothes lines.

Frigidity: sexual impotence in females. Includes the failure to achieve orgasm during the sexual act.

Homosexuality: attraction towards persons of the same sex or of both sexes (bisexuality).

Impotence: difficulty in carrying out the sexual act. The problem may be premature ejaculation or inability to obtain or sustain an errection. The cause is usually psychological.

Lesbian: the term used to describe a female homosexual.

Masochism: obtaining of sexual pleasure from being beaten and hurt – pain pleasure.

Necrophily: sexual gratification from dead bodies.

Paedophilia: sexual passion for children.

Sadism: obtaining of sexual pleasure from inflicting pain on a partner.

Transvestism: obtaining of sexual pleasure and orgasm from dressing in the clothes of the opposite sex.

Voyeurism: obtaining of pleasure from watching other people undress or take part in sexual activities – 'Peeping Toms'.

Sexual Disorders – treatment of: many sexually disordered patients are embarrassed and some never ask for treatment. Behaviour therapy, desensitisation and aversion therapy may help, also psychotherapy in some cases. Consultation with a sex therapist may be useful.

Sibling: offspring of the same mother – brothers and sisters.

Somnambulism: sleep-walking.

Soporific: any sleep-inducing agent.

Stereotypy: the constant repetition of an action e.g. constantly rubbing some part of the body.

Sterilisation: the process of causing a person to become sterile, to render conception impossible.

Strabismus: eye squint.

Suggestion: the process of encouraging a person to accept uncritically an idea or belief.

Super-ego: in psychoanalytical psychology the super-ego is an unconscious part of the mind which has the following functions:

    (a) Sets moral standards for the ego (right and wrong)

    (b) Controls primitive demands of the id

    (c) Promotes critical self-observation

    (d) Inflicts self-punishment

Tabes: wasting. Tabes dorsalis is a chronic disease of the nervous system due to syphilis.

Twilight State: disturbance in consciousness with diminished awareness during which the patient may carry out purposeless acts with no subsequent memory for them e.g. in hysteria; post epileptic fit.

Vasectomy: a sterilising operation on men whereby the seminal ducts are cut and tied off.

Wilson, S. A. K.: English neurologist. Wilson's disease is characterised by tetanoid chorea. The involuntary laughing and rigidity are similar to those seen in Parkinsonism; a hereditary disorder of copper metabolism causing degeneration of the corpus striatum and cirrhosis of the liver.

Psychology

Adolescence: the term used to describe the period following puberty, the teen years from 12–18. A period of rapid growth and development when the secondary sexual characteristics develop. Adolescents may be self-conscious of their physical development. There is a development of interest in the opposite sex, an identification with peer groups and youth culture, new mental energy and individualism, striving for freedom and recognition, rebelliousness against parents and teachers. Further education and career decisions must be made. Inferiority, inadequacy and boredom may be problems.

Adulthood: in law a person is an adult at 18 years. Adulthood consolidates during the 'twenties'. This is a period of continuing maturity and personality integration; career development; courtship, marriage, building a home, parenthood and raising a family.

Age, Mental (MA): related to intelligence measurement. The age at which an individual is functioning intellectually as compared with the average. For example, an average 7 year old child has an MA of 7 but if his performance in an intelligence test is the same as an 9 year old boy, he would have a MA of 9.

Age, Middle: the period from approximately 45 – 55 years. This may be a period of contentment and stability but is also a potentially dangerous time. Children are now grown up, there is more time to think, brood on failed ambitions, to fear illness and death, or to worry over sexual and physical attractiveness, adjusting to the physiological changes associated with the menopause and so on. Depression and anxiety may occur.

Age, Old: physiological ageing is shown by slower movements, stiffness, wrinkling skin, faulty hearing and vision, brittle bones and tooth decay. Mental ageing may show as slight intellectual decline, memory absences, stubbornness, independence, suspicion, anxiety, confusion and depression.

Anger: unpleasant emotion, unfriendly feeling. Anger may be displayed by shouting, screaming, quarrelling and physical blows.

Attitude: a favourable or unfavourable way of feeling, acting or thinking in relation to some person or thing. It is an opinion ultimately determined by feeling and not intellect (Spencer). Attitudes help us to react quickly e.g. views relating to politics, religion, football, etc. Important attitudes in nurses include: tolerance, understanding, patience, honesty, reliability, pride, punctuality and integrity.

Childhood (1 – 5 years): physical development in the second year of life is concerned with walking, talking, and toilet training.

Play and parental encouragement are important for physical development. During the second year the child's memory is developing or recollection is possible, though development in the pre-school child consists of egocentric thinking and his speech is usually a running commentary on his thoughts. Children in this age group have no regard for another's point of view and everything is black and white, up and down, right and left, with little flexibility. Security, interest, love and affection from the parents are essential for a healthy development.

Childhood (5 – 12 years): school marks the first major break from the home and introduces the child to the wider society. Concrete learning can commence at 7 years, (primary school) and abstract learning usually commences at 11 – 12 years (secondary education). Play becomes less individual and more group and gang organised.

Emotion: affect; feeling. Emotions are mostly inherited and make us respond in a certain way (e.g. fear, anger, love and hate). Some emotions are pleasant, some are unpleasant. Moods are longer-lasting emotions. Expression of emotion may bring body changes e.g. behaviour (running), muscular (trembling) and circulatory (pallor).

Extrovert: a person with outward looking personality who prefers action to thought, and company to being alone.

Eysenck, H. J.: British psychologist who developed the three dimensional personality theory. He holds controversial views on intelligence, (i.e. intelligence is mostly inherited and may be linked to social class and race) and is an advocate of behavioural therapy and objective personality tests.

Fixation: remaining at an early stage of psychological development.

Gesell, Arnold: American psychologist who suggested norms for development in infancy, e.g. at 28 weeks a baby begins to articulate sounds, at 52 weeks he should crawl about freely and at 78 weeks bladder control should be established during the day.

Groups, Psychological: a group, in psychological terms, is a number of people who get together for a common purpose and interest. Groups are used to treat patients with mental illness (i.e. therapeutic groups e.g. group therapy).

Groups, Social: Groups are social systems in which people interact and are found in all societies e.g. family groups, peer groups, political groups, religious groups.

Id: the deep and unconscious part of the mind.

Infancy: the period of development from 0–1 year when an infant is dependent on mothering for his needs. Bowlby states that infants need a warm, intimate and continuous relationship with the mother.

Instincts: patterns of behaviour that are biologically inherited and do not need learning e.g. sucking, sex, hunger, maternalism. Not all psychologists agree on the inheritance aspect of instincts.

Intelligence: the ability to think rationally, learn, reason and form concepts. Psychologists disagree on the nature of intelligence but it is generally accepted that both inherited and environmental factors are important.

Intelligence Quotient (IQ): intelligence test scores; the ratio of mental age over real age × 100.

Learning: acquiring new skills and responses; gaining knowledge and understanding of our perceptions.

Learning, Insightful: involves learning by insight, looking at the problem, studying it and then solving it. Aimless activity is reduced by knowing in advance what action to take.

Learning, Trial and Error: learning from wrong actions and mistakes.

Maternal Deprivation: lack of mothering; neglect of child by mother. In 1951, John Bowlby published the results of research on maternal deprivation: it can be the cause of delinquency, psychiatric distress and other psychiatric illnesses in later years. Mother love in infancy and childhood is as important for mental health as vitamins and protein for physical health. Bowlby's research has gained wide acceptance but not all psychologists agree, e.g. Casler (1968) states 'The human organism does not need maternal love in order to function normally'.

Maturity: Functioning and physical completeness. Maturity is often elusive because the more mature a person's behaviour is, the more likely he is to be aware of his inadequacies. Intelligence reaches maturity at 16 years. Physical maturity in terms of growth is reached by 18 years. Emotional maturity is the ability to control emotional responses and display emotions in a socially acceptable way; some people never achieve this.

Mental Mechanisms (personality defence mechanism): in psychodynamics theories (such as those of Freud) certain facesaving defence mechanisms are considered important. These are processes which happen when we are under stress or conflict and no constructive solution of our problem can be found. In these circumstances we use mental mechanisms to protect ourselves, save face, cover up, readjust or preserve our self-esteem. The important mental mechanisms are listed below:

Conversion: when an anxiety or dissociation takes a physical form such as paralysis or blindness.

Displacement: the unconscious movement of feelings produced by one object to another more convenient object, (taking it out on something else e.g. kicking the dog, banging the door).

Dissociation: the separation of experiences from one, other in the mind. An experience is locked away in the mind e.g. loss of memory in hysteria.

Projection: when a person's faults and weaknesses are seen as being present in other people rather than the person himself, e.g., relatives may unconsciously feel responsible for the patient's illness but may accuse the hospital staff of neglect.

Rationalisation: (self-deception): giving logical and rational excuses after the event so as to justify your situation e.g. 'I didn't get the job because my face doesn't fit.'

Reaction Formation: when the opposite is true regarding feelings or behaviour e.g. 'I am inferior to you' becomes 'I am superior to you'.

Regression: going back to behaviour applicable to an earlier period of development (e.g. child-like dependency on others and childish approach to problems).

Repression: the unconscious forgetting of something unpleasant e.g. a dental appointment.

Sublimation: substituting something else which is socially acceptable e.g. a woman who is unable to find satisfaction in marriage may take up charity work.

Suppression: the conscious forgetting of feelings or wishes.

Motivation: human motivation is concerned with the drive and energy. An individual displays motive, power of thought and action. Freudian psychology implies that motivation may be influenced by unconscious repression, (e.g. sex and aggression). Marx's philosophy implies that the main motive to work is money and control of capital and production.

Perception: the awareness and interpretation by the brain of stimuli from our sense organs — the way we take things in and give them a meaning. Previous experience, emotions and personality may influence our perceptions.

Perception Errors: persons may be subjected to the same stimuli but interpret them differently. Patients with faulty sense organs may make perceptual errors (e.g. elderly patients). Illusions are perceptual errors. Attention and observation reduce errors.

Personality: involves the whole person in terms of their characteristics, interests, attributes, traits and so on. Two terms may be used in relation to personality: (a) temperament, which is a person's habitual mental outlook or the way they look at life (such as optimistic and pessimistic) and (b) character, which relates to a person's qualities, attitudes and behaviour (such as honesty and reliability).

Prejudice: an unfavourable attitude which is based on a rigid and irrational view which is usually contrary to facts.

Puberty: the period of development which marks the physical changes from childhood to manhood and womanhood. (The age of puberty onset varies e.g. some girls may reach puberty at 11 years but others may be as late as 15 years.) The age when a person becomes capable of sexual reproduction.

Retention: information which is learnt is stored by the brain. When we remember something the memory is reactivated and brought into our consciousness (recall). Forgetting is a failure to recall; the passage of time makes recall more difficult.

Sociology

Achieved Status: a status one works for; a social position achieved through effort rather than birthright.

Alienation: separation from certain social conditions; e.g. workers isolated from management – no control over the means of production may give workers a sense of powerlessness.

Ascribed Status: a status or social position obtained by birthright; inherited status.

Authority: the legitimate power to make others act in some way on bureaucratic, traditional or charismatic grounds (Weber).

Bureaucracy: an ideal type of administrative organisation; 'red tape'. Includes hierarchy of offices with spheres of competency, systematic promotion. Acts and decisions are recorded in minutes, staff are salary paid and no one individual is indispensable.

Class: a position or ranking in the community based on factors such as income, roots, occupation, and neighbourhood: working class, middle class, upper class.

Deliquency: minor criminal acts; petty crime among young persons (delinquents).

Division of Labour: the division of work into a number of parts with each part being done by a separate individual or group; assembly line work.

Embourgeoisement: the theory that the lines between social classes are becoming more blurred.

Extended Family: a married couple and their children together with direct relatives.

Nuclear Family: a close family unit of husband, wife and children.

Peer Group: a group of members from one's own age group.

Pressure Group: a group of persons with similar goals who strive to influence decision making.

Profession: an occupational group which demands special knowledge and skills for membership.

Role: the part one plays in a particular social setting.

Role-expectation: how the role player and others see a person's role.

Social Norms: the standards shared by group members to which individuals conform.

Socialisation: the process whereby we learn the rules and practices of social groups; the transmission of culture from the previous generation to the present.

Recommended Reading List
and Guide to Content

* denotes an out of print book. These texts have been included where
they are helpful and relevant reading for the student, and should be
obtained through libraries.

1 Basic books on psychiatry

Dally, P. J. 1982. *Psychology and Psychiatry*. (5th edition), Hodder
and Stoughton, Sevenoaks.
Gives a basic account of psychology and psychiatry including
management and treatment.
Gibson, J. 1979. *Psychiatry for Nurses*, (4th edition). Blackwell
Scientific, Oxford.
A guide to mental disorders, clinical descriptions and
treatments.
Koshy, K. T. 1982. *Revision Notes on Psychiatry*, (2nd edition).
Hodder and Stoughton, Sevenoaks.
A short condensed text on basic psychiatry.
Watkins, M. 1983. *Multiple Choice Questions: Psychiatry*. Hodder
& Stoughton, Sevenoaks.
400 questions and answers with explanations covering psy-
chology, communication, psychiatry, nursing care and prac-
tice. Useful for learning and revision.

2 Intermediate depth books on psychiatry

Curran, D., Partridge, M. A., and Storey, P. B. 1980. *Psychological
Medicine*, (9th edition). Churchill Livingstone, Edinburgh.
Comprehensive psychiatry and treatment.
Sainsbury, M. J. 1980. *Key to Psychiatry*, (3rd edition). Harvey,
Miller and Metcalf, Aylesbury.
Comprehensive psychiatry including accounts of therapeutic
team management and the psychiatric nurse's role

3 In-depth and reference books

Henderson, D. K. and Gillespie, R. D. 1969. *Textbook of
Psychiatry*, (10th edition). Oxford Medical, Oxford. In-depth
psychiatry including case discussion and treatment

4 Specific (specialist) books and publications

Bird, J., Marks, I. M. and Lindley, P. 1979. 'Nurse therapists in psychiatry: Developments, controversies and implications'. *British Journal of Psychiatry*, Oct., 321–29.

Butler, R. J. and Rosenthal, G. 1978. *Behaviour and Rehabilitation.* John Wright, Bristol.
Outlines the procedures involved in behaviour modification with long term patients.

Carr, P. J. and others, 1979. *Community Psychiatric Nursing.* Churchill Livingstone, Edinburgh.
Clearly describes the principles and aims underlying the community psychiatric services.

Craft, M. 1966. *Psychopathic Disorders and their Assessment.* Pergamon Press, Oxford.
A textbook on psychopathy and its management.

Crisp, A. H. 1976. *British Journal of Psychiatry*, **128**, 549–54.

Dally, P. J. 1979. *Anorexia Nervosa.* Heineman Medical Books, London.

Gillis, L. 1980. *Human Behaviour in Illness.* Faber and Faber, London.
An account of how behaviour is affected by illness and hospitalisation.

Greenland, C. 1970. *Mental Health and Civil Liberty.* Occasional Paper on Social Administration, No. 38. Bell & Hyman, London.
A study of Mental Health Review Tribunals in England and Wales.

Guidelines for the care of patients undergoing electroconvulsive therapy. 1982, Royal College of Nursing, London.

Heaton-Ward, W. A. 1975. *Mental Sub-normality*, (4th edition). John Wright and Sons, Bristol.
An account of mental handicap conditions and their treatment and care.

Hodkinson, M. 1966. *Nursing the Elderly.* Pergamon Press, Oxford.
Nursing care of the elderly and associated disorders.

International Classification of Diseases. 1967. World Health Organisation, Geneva.

Marks, I. M. *et al.* 1978. *Nursing in Behavioural Psychotherapy.* Churchill Livingstone, Edinburgh.
The role of the psychiatric nurse as a therapist.

Merchant, O. O. 1981. 'Reality Orientation—A Way Forward'. *Nursing Times*, **77**, 1442–1445.

* Mitchell, R. 1974. *Advances in Psychiatry*. Macmillan Journals, London.
  A collection of essays on mental illness and views on treatment concepts.
* Pryse-Phillips, W. 1969. *Epilepsy*. John Wright and Sons, Bristol.
  Specific text on epilepsy and treatment.
Roberts, N. 1967. *Mental Health and Mental Illness*. Routledge and Kegan Paul, London.
  Past and modern history of psychiatry including future plans and trends in the care of the mentally ill.
Franks, C. M. and Rubin, R. D. (Eds). 1969. *Advances in Behaviour Therapy*, **Vol. 1.** Academic Press, London.
  An account of behavioural therapy and its application to psychiatric conditions.
* Willis, J. 1969. *Drug Dependence*. Faber and Faber, London.
  A text on drug dependence and its treatment.
* Wolf, S. and Wolf, H. E. 1947. *Human Gastric Function*. Oxford University Press, Oxford and New York.
Wolpe, J. 1982. *The Practice of Behaviour Therapy*. (3rd edition) Pergamon, New York and Oxford.
Zangwill, O. L. 1980. *Report of the Joint Working Party on Behaviour Modification*. HMSO, London.

5 Social skills and communication

Argyle, M. 1983. *The Psychology of Interpersonal Behaviour*. (4th edition) Penguin Books, Harmondsworth.
Gahagan, J. 1975. *Interpersonal and Group Behaviour*. Methuen, London.
* Paplau, H. E. 1952. *Interpersonal Relations in Nursing*. Putnam & Co., New York.
Ruesch, J. 1967. *The Human Dialogue*. Free Press, New York.
Trower, P. and others 1978. *Social Skills and Mental Health*. Methuen, London.

6 Other books and publications

Barton, R. 1976. *Institutional Neurosis*, (3rd edition) John Wright and Sons, Bristol.
Eysenck, H. J. 1975. *The Future of Psychiatry*. Methuen, London.
Franklin, B. 1975. *The Study of Nursing Care*, Series 1 No. 5. Ron Publications, London.

Goffman, E. 1970. *Asylums.* Penguin Books, Harmondsworth.

Jones, M. 1968. *Beyond the Therapeutic Community.* Yale University Press, New Haven, Conn.

Laing, R. D. 1970. *The Divided Self.* Penguin Books, Harmondsworth.

Laing, R. D. and Esterson, A. 1970, *Sanity, Madness and the Family*, **Vol. 1.** Penguin Books, Harmondsworth.

Szasz, T. S. 1973. *The Manufacture of Madness.* Paladin, London.

Szasz, T. S. 1976. *The Myth of Mental Illness.* Harper and Row, New York.

Szasz, T. S. 1975. *The Age of Madness.* Routledge, London.

Index

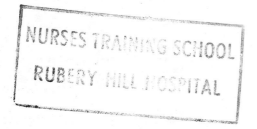